# THE WOMAN'S HOLISTIC HEADACHE RELIEF BOOK

JUNE BIERMANN & BARBARA TOOHEY

J. P. Tarcher, Inc.
Los Angeles
Distributed by St. Martin's Press
New York

*To Martha Kuljian,*
*the only person who ever sent June a get-well card*
*during her entire five years of chronic headaches*

Library of Congress Catalog Card No. 78-62793
Distributor's ISBN: 0-312-90971-3
Publisher's ISBN: 0-87477-086-6

Illustrated by Adrienne Picchi
Design: John Brogna
Manufactured in the United States of America

Published by J. P. Tarcher, Inc.
9110 Sunset Blvd., Los Angeles, Calif. 90069
Published simultaneously in Canada by Macmillan of Canada
70 Bond St., Toronto, Canada M5B 1X3

# CONTENTS

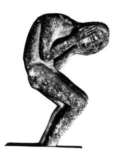

*La Damnée*, detail from tympan, Autun Cathedral, France

*I am very brave generally . . . only today I happen to have a headache.*

Lewis Carroll
*Through the Looking Glass*

# FOREWORD

A patient with headaches deserves compassion, understanding, and a holistic approach in the best sense of
the word.

Headaches cannot be objectively measured. Physicians,
family, friends, and co-workers can, therefore, choose to
ignore or misinterpret headaches. This adds to the patient's
distress and depression, which in turn aggravate the
headache. Headaches can be very severe. They can be dis-
abling. They can destroy a person's coping mechanism and
self-esteem. They can destroy marriages and other inter-
personal relationships. They can lead to suicidal depression. They often lead to desperate attempts by the headache
sufferer to find a cure. In the process, he or she may face
financial ruin. Often, a headache patient is referred to a
psychiatrist whose chances of success are generally just as
limited as those of his medical colleagues.

In most patients, headaches are the result of a multitude
of contributing factors arising from both lifestyle and phys-

ical conditions. It is not unusual for a difficult case to be seen by many different specialists. The important consideration is that all these health professionals be interested in headaches and highly skilled and that the effort be well coordinated.

This book describes the above situations and offers practical information on diagnosis and treatment of headaches in an understandable and positive manner. It is filled with the excitement of a "detective story" that unravels at a quick pace the mystery of a case of severe recurrent headaches. I read this book with fascination in one uninterrupted session. I read it with a smile and many chuckles, and with admiration for the authors, who have accumulated such a wealth of information and advice.

Although this is called *The Woman's Holistic Headache Relief Book*, it is actually a book for both women *and* men, for both patients *and* doctors, and for all those who experience life as an endless struggle to create and maintain a positive balance of forces in the midst of the misery and despair of headaches.

Gunnar Heuser, M.D., Ph.D., F.A.C.P.
Beverly Hills Headache and Pain
Medical Group

# ACKNOWLEDGMENTS

Since June's headache mystery had such an all-star cast, we would like to thank them in alphabetical order.

Otto Appenzeller, M.D., Ph.D., who removed the Achilles heel from our running section.

Frances Hardy Boston, who first discovered Dr. Heuser for us — to our minds, a medical discovery second only to the discovery of radium.

Mark Brim, D.P.M., who showed us that when it comes to pain, the foot bone can be connected to the head bone.

David Bresler, Ph.D., who deserves a four-hug salute for his lucid explanations of holistic principles.

Janice Gallagher, our editor, whose attention to detail, indomitable sense of humor, and fighting spirit saved the day — and the book.

Jack Gariss, whose KPFK radio broadcasts first turned June's mind Eastward.

Arnold Greene, D.D.S., who had the confidence he could cure June's headaches and the skill to do it.

Helen Herman, Valley College Headache Underground member and librarian, who brought her pain and her profession to the reading of our manuscript.

Gunnar Heuser, M.D., Ph.D., F.A.C.P., without whom there would have been no book — and maybe by now, no June.

Albert P. Krueger, M.D., who showed us the positive effects negative ions can have on headaches.

Charles Ledergerber, M.D., and Mirjam Ledergerber, who wanted to make a contribution to their adopted country and *have*.

Dorothy Lindholm, the right hemisphere of the Beverly Hills Headache and Pain Medical Group, who had endless tolerance for our endless questions and became our newest old friend.

Victor Mintz, D.D.S., scholar and raconteur, who jawboned us through the final draft of our TMJ section.

Douglas Morgan, D.D.S., who with his patience and patients gave us new insights into TMJ diagnosis and therapy.

Gerald Pearlman, D.C., who adjusted — among other things — our thinking about headaches.

Penny Pollard, Valley College Headache Underground member, who shared the continuing saga of her headache cure with us.

Linda Sharp, exercise therapist, who stretched our minds with information on exorcising pain through exercise.

Shannon Stack, Ph.D., Valley College Headache Underground member, who gave June Cafergot and sympathy.

Emile White, Valley College Headache Underground member, who made biofeedback palatable for us.

And, finally, Barbara would like to thank June for continually getting health problems for us to write about and June would like to thank Barbara for never giving up until we have them solved.

# INTRODUCTION
---
# TWO HEADS,
# ONE HEADACHE

$R$adio and TV talk show hosts have a favorite opening gambit when interviewing authors. They always ask, "Why did you write this book?" Sometimes it's a tough question to answer, but in this case it's easy. We wrote this book on headaches because we desperately needed it ourselves; June as a firsthand sufferer and Barbara as her writing collaborator who became a secondhand victim of the pain. As a matter of fact, in the last few years we've written all of our books as much for ourselves as for others.

In the early days of our eighteen-year writing collaboration we specialized in humor and satire, in fun and games, writing books and articles on such subjects as gourmet dining and wining, foreign travel, skiing, and bicycling. Then suddenly the fun was over when about ten years ago the June-half of our partnership discovered she had diabetes. Barbara felt almost as if she, too, had been condemned with the affliction because when your collaborator is out of whack it's like having half the keys on your typewriter busted.

Since we're both librarians at Los Angeles Valley College, as well as writers, we have great faith in the power of the printed word. We prowled libraries throughout Southern California, reading everything we could find on the subject of diabetes, trying to discover how June could resume her active, freewheeling way of living despite her disease. No luck. Everything we read made it sound as if she'd have to spend the rest of her days living like a laboratory rat. We couldn't accept this death sentence on both the good life for June and the continued existence of the collaboration, so we started experimenting and learning. Eventually June overcame the handicap that diabetes is thought to be. Then, drawing from our research and diabetic adventures and misadventures, we wrote a guidebook to good health and good times for diabetics, *The Peripatetic Diabetic*. Later we followed it up with *The Diabetes Question and Answer Book* and *The Diabetic's Sports and Exercise Book*.

June's life was beautiful again. The collaboration flourished, toting up ten books and over three hundred magazine articles. Then June, who could be called the woman who has everything, was suddenly zapped once more. This time it was chronic headaches. Intense and incapacitating and virtually insupportable, they pounded away in her skull one third of her waking hours and occupied all of her should-be working mind.

In an attempt to cure them, besides consulting specialist after specialist who prescribed drug after drug, we turned again to the library for aid and comfort. There we found a number of books on headaches, most written by doctors, none dealing specifically with the unique problems of women, and all virtually worthless to the sufferer. The book jackets promised they were going to tell how to get relief from headaches. The pages inside broke the promise. The main concern was always to pin a label on the headache—"tension," "allergy," "cluster," "sinus," and that great catchall, "migraine." After helping the sufferer label herself—usually incorrectly—they seemed to feel their responsibility was over, leaving her as miserable as ever. After all, a headache by any name hurts just as much.

Sometimes the doctor-authors treated the reader to case histories of their more brilliant diagnoses. A favorite of these case histories was the discovery that the patient was a Chinese food freak and that the monosodium glutamate in Oriental food was causing headaches. June read that one so many times that she can still hardly look a plate of egg foo yung in the eye without a feeling of nausea.

Oh yes, there were also the "great medical breakthrough" articles that you fall upon when you're in line at the supermarket and the *National Enquirer* screeches at you with headlines like, "NEW MIRACLE CURE FOR HEADACHES."

June tried every idea she read. When you're desperate, you'll try anything. If someone had told her that her headaches would go away if she smeared bat guano in her hair and marched nude down Hollywood Boulevard by the light of the full moon, she probably would have done it. And it probably would have done her as much good as the rest of the "miracle cures."

No, the written word failed us again. Once more we had to fight it out for ourselves. With luck and pluck and the determination of two desperate women we finally won our victory over June's pain.

You may think you don't have a chance for such a victory since you're struggling by yourself without the advantages of a concerned collaborator-friend and of a background in medical research. You're wrong. You are no longer alone. You have us. You now have the advantage of *two* concerned collaborator-friends with backgrounds in medical research.

We've gathered up all of our five years of library investigation, our exciting discoveries about holism, and our experience (which, as Oscar Wilde said, is the name we give to our mistakes). With this material we wrote the book June needed, the book we searched for in vain when she was first felled by headaches, the book you need now.

Although our motivation here is the same as with our books on June's other chronic condition, diabetes, our goal is slightly different. With those we wanted to show the reader how to live happily ever after with diabetes; with this book we want to show you how to live happily ever after *without* headaches.

# PART ONE

## A HOLISTIC APPROACH TO YOUR HEADACHES: SEARCHING FOR CLUES

# 1

# THE HISTORY OF YOUR HEADACHE

Feminist claims to the contrary, God is definitely *not* a woman. We have evidence. A female God would never have designed human bodies so that a man can eat 10 percent more calories than a woman and not gain weight. She wouldn't have bestowed upon us all the cramps and inconveniences of menstruation and the vagaries of menopause. She wouldn't have subjected us to the ever-present fear of rape. But the greatest proof of all is that She wouldn't have arranged for Her sisters to suffer the lioness's share of headaches.

The United States leads the world in headaches with an estimated 45 million chronic sufferers. In New York City alone ten thousand aspirins are swallowed every minute of the day. And it's fairly certain that 85 percent of those that are consumed for headaches are going down *female* gullets, since 85 percent of America's regular headache victims are women.

Why this disproportionate percentage of women? Female hormonal balances enter into it, but they aren't the whole story. We feel the demands of a woman's life are even more significant. Like any cliché, "a woman's work is never done" has a lot of truth in it. We women tend to feel responsible for everything and everybody for every minute of every day. As one woman put it, "No matter what I'm doing at any given moment, I feel guilty because I'm not doing something else."

The pressure builds. The headache fastens on, and because a woman feels she has to keep functioning at all costs, she begs from the doctor or borrows from a sister sufferer a pain killer, a tranquilizer, anything to help her get through her day, her life. No wonder that 85 percent of the headache sufferers are women.

And of the 85 percent, all have at one time or another been dismissed as whining neurotics. There's an old saying among male medical professionals that "men describe their symptoms," while "women complain." Some doctors even hate to see a woman suffering from chronic headaches enter their offices. Among themselves they refer to these patients as "crocks," medical slang for hypochondriacs and malingerers. Another popular dismissal they have for the mature woman with chronic headaches is, "She just has the FFF syndrome—female, fat, and forty."

No, headache victims are not favorites of physicians, probably because they have no idea of how to help them. These doctors fail mainly because they seek the one-and-only cause of a patient's headaches when, in reality, they are caused by a multiplicity of factors. We discovered that the holistically oriented doctor who deals with a patient's total physical and mental condition as well as her lifestyle and environment can more effectively diagnose, treat, and cure headaches. Unfortunately, the holistic medical approach to headaches is not widespread in the medical community where both holism and headaches have not received serious consideration until recently. It is, in fact, only within the last decade that headaches and chronic pain have been recognized by the medical profession as treatable conditions in themselves and not just neuroses to be referred to psychiatrists or symptoms to be numbed with drugs.

One of the reasons there has been so little real concern and help for sufferers is that no one actually dies of a headache, although those afflicted with them often entertain the idea of death as the only possible release from their agony. A. Alvarez, in his book *The Savage God*, mentions an increase in poet Sylvia Plath's sinus headaches as one of the devastating life factors that combined to draw her head into the oven. Indeed, one specialist speaking at a headache seminar we attended mentioned that he had lost only two headache patients in his career—both from a bullet through the brain. It is a wonder more women (and men, too, for that matter) don't take this extreme route out of pain and frustration.

In the beginning the headache sufferer has hope for alleviation and a cure, but before long she becomes a medical orphan knocking on one specialist's door after another, trying to find a haven from her pain. She comes to feel that most of her time is spent holding her head in doctors' waiting rooms. She writes check after check for what prove to be worthless tests and treatments, eventually developing an understandable distrust and hostility toward the medical profession. Almost inevitably she comes to the point where her money and hope run out and so do those commodities even more important to her sanity and survival: the sympathy and understanding of her family members, friends, and colleagues. Everyone becomes bored with her constant complaints because they don't really think of her as being sick. After all, *everybody* has headaches at one time or another.

As the recurrent headaches continue month after month and year after year, the sufferer accumulates more and more mental problems—depression, anxiety, and, in extreme cases, personality deterioration and suicidal impulses. (It is not surprising that among chronic headache sufferers the divorce rate runs from 60 to 80 percent.) The end result is that she becomes what you might call a "headachoholic," not in the sense that she *needs* her headaches (although some women actually do without realizing it), but rather in the sense that she is dominated, controlled, and virtually destroyed by headaches, even as alcoholics are by alcohol. But, although headache sufferers outnumber alcoholics five to one, they don't get nearly the attention that drinkers do. As we researched this book at the UCLA Biomedical Library, we discovered that this major scientific collection contained over three hundred books on alcoholism and only about thirty on headaches.

We've been rehashing all these dismals for you, not out of sadistic impulses but rather to show you that from both personal and peripheral experience we know what the anguish of chronic headache suffering is. We do not, like most doctors, deal with the problem as outsiders.

From our inside experience of having lived through June's five-year season in the headache jungle and having finally hacked our way out of it, we are certain that we can show you, too, how to diminish your pain and force it to release its hammerlock on your life. No matter how long you've had your pain—if you've had it for six months or more we consider it chronic—or how many "cures" you've tried or whether you've been to one or one hundred doctors, we can offer you new ideas and great expectations. You don't have to resign yourself to learning to live with three-quarter time, half-time, or quarter-time headache pain. We are convinced that whether you have what you consider a major, a middling, or a minor chronic headache problem, you can do something about it. We even believe that many of you, like June, can give yourself more than relief. You can discover a permanent cure for your headaches.

## THE HOLISTIC APPROACH

How are we going to lead you out of your personal headache jungle? The word "holistic" in the title of this book indicates the path we're going to take. Holistic healing is different from conventional Western medicine. In holistic medicine the body and the mind are considered inseparable, an idea Eastern healers have recognized for centuries; while Western medicine has traditionally divided illness into two distinct categories, physical and mental. And to complete this sense of wholeness, your body, mind, and spirit are seen in the entire context of your world—your relationships, your lifestyle, and your environment. (As we heard a holistically inclined internist lament, "If only we could treat the patient's surroundings.") Holistic medicine thus emphasizes treating you as a whole rather than as a collection of body parts functioning independently. (The word holistic is sometimes spelled "*w*holistic.")

Yet another concept of holism is its emphasis on wellness rather than on illness. We find this a particularly apt approach for headache sufferers who, after months or years of misery, tend to accept pain as their natural state and to program themselves for feeling bad instead of for feeling good. If, on the other hand, they could watch for and reward themselves for positive feelings, they could change their outlook on their pain and perhaps eventually eliminate it.

But there's an even more important value in holistic healing, especially for headache sufferers. Holistic physicians and practitioners teach a different attitude toward sickness and pain. They teach that each of us has a major role as a self-healer participating in our own cure. In going to doctors and taking advantage of the latest medical treatments you do not passively hand yourself over to a physician to do with you what he will. (We say "he," and will do so throughout, because almost all physicians who specialize in headache treatment in the U.S. are male.) Yes, the doctor is there, but as your helper, your therapist, or, as we like to think of him, your collaborator. As a full partner in your treatment you have opinions and make decisions. You monitor your own body sensations and reactions. In short, you not only participate in the alleviation or cure, but you are also ultimately responsible for it. Just as war is too important to be left to the generals, your health is too important to be left to the doctors.

Playing a leading role in your own cure and tracking down just what in the "whole" of your life is causing your headaches is complex detective work. And as Sir Robert Mark, the recently retired head of Scotland Yard, put it, "Good detective work takes a combination of brains, logic, and perseverance." To help you develop this winning combination we're first going to show you, by way of both positive and negative example, the detective work we did to solve the mystery of June's headache problem. (You will notice that much of the time, rather than operating with Scotland Yard skill, we were blundering around like Inspector Clouseau, eagerly following the wrong clues, inadvertently destroying evidence.) Then we're going to help you write your own unique headache mystery story and track down and record clues in a much more efficient, direct, and intelligent manner than we did with June's case. And finally we're going to lead you through relief measures and body-mind techniques that may alleviate the complex problems that are causing your headaches. Should you still require some detection help, we'll put you on the trail of the holistic doctor. Finally, we offer you some encouragement as you start on the road to recovery. Let us begin, then, with the Curious Case of the Chronic Headache.

# 2

## JUNE'S MYSTERY HEADACHE

If you like exotic settings for the openings of mystery stories, we have one for you: the Far West Ski Association charter flight from Geneva to Los Angeles. Not quite the Orient Express, but at least an international means of transportation.

We were returning home from a working vacation of skiing and gathering material for articles on Alpine ski resorts. June, crammed into the narrow charter-size seat, looked something less than prime—bleary of eye and drippy of nose from a cold she picked up a week before in Cortina, Italy—and the thirteen-hour flight didn't help.

The first day home June felt worse. There was a weakness, a fever, and a lead-boned feeling associated with that year's imported flu. And there was one more symptom: a headache. It was a pain behind the bridge of the nose and the eyeballs, and it radiated into the forehead.

This was an unfamiliar pain to June. She wasn't a headache person. In fact, during her first forty years she

9

had never had a headache except during her only two hangovers: one mild, one a doozie.

Gradually the rest of her symptoms went away but the headache lingered, changing from a minor irritation ("I'll be glad when I get rid of this headache.") to a major preoccupation ("Isn't this damned headache *ever* going away?"). But June never really doubted that it *would* go away.

When she visited her internist for her regular diabetes check-up, the headache had been hanging on for a month. In the discussion period following the examination June complained, "Ever since I got the flu I've had this headache that won't go away." When the doctor asked if she'd been under any unusual stress, her dry response was, "No, only the usual stress of juggling two careers and living with diabetes plus the stress these headaches are causing."

June's internist whipped out his speculum, peered up her nose, hmmmmmmmmmmed, and said her sinuses were swollen. And since a major function of an internist is to point the patient toward a specialist, he pointed to an ENT—an ear, nose, and throat man—or, as they're known in medical circles, an otolaryngologist.

## THE TIME OF THE SINUSES

June dutifully followed the point that lead to an office almost as crowded as the Tokyo subway at rush hour. After about an hour-and-a-half wait, she got to see the doctor, who turned off the lights and gave her transillumination. Although this may sound like a mystical religious experience, it just means putting a patient in a darkened room and flashing a light over the sinus areas. After the obligatory medical hmmmmmmmmmm, he seconded the internist's diagnosis of swollen sinuses. Infected ethmoids, to be specific. He had his nurse irrigate June's sinuses by sticking a small rubber tube in one nostril and running a solution through it, up into the sinuses and out the other nostril—a treatment June came to loathe and refer to as "the old hose-in-the-nose." After being presented with a prescription for an antibiotic and a bill, she was sent on her way.

June had the headache for a couple more days, and then it drifted away. Since she dislikes contaminating her body with any drug except your basic caffeine and alcohol, she stopped taking the antibiotic, figuring that was that—the end of an unpleasant but mercifully short chapter in her book of health.

But then one morning a few weeks later she awoke to find that the headache had clamped on again. It was the same sharp bridge-of-nose–eyeball pain radiating to the forehead that gradually settled into a dull, unremitting ache.

In the two weeks before she could get another appointment with the otolaryngologist, she had on/again, off/again, mostly on/again headaches. The doctor was still convinced it was an infection of the ethmoid sinuses. The problem was, he explained, that she had stopped taking the antibiotic too soon. She was supposed to have taken all the medicine prescribed and shouldn't have quit just because the symptoms went away.

June resumed taking the antibiotic. There was some remission of pain, but the off-and-on headaches continued. She was beginning to lose patience. So was Barbara. Our collaboration was starting to suffer from headaches. We could get no work done because we were always discussing them. "Do you have one now?" "How long have you had it this time?" "Is it getting any better?" "You've got to get that doctor to do something about it!"

We both felt that the doctor just hadn't pressed the right button and that there *was* a button to press. Another appointment with the doctor, another hour-and-a-half wait, another hose-in-the-nose, another antibiotic prescription, but still the headaches continued, switching on and off with the regularity of a neon sign.

Discouraged with the otolaryngologist, we decided to try to figure out for ourselves what was wrong. After all, with three diabetes books under our belts we considered ourselves medical experts of a sort, and as librarians we certainly knew how to do research. We set about methodically reading every section of every book in the Valley College library that dealt with sinus trouble and headaches. We uncovered the information that usually with a sinus infection there is a discharge of mucus. June had never had a discharge. Not only that, but we also learned that sinus trouble is a fairly uncommon cause of chronic headaches, TV commercial claims to the contrary. Finally, we read that it is impossible to see the ethmoid sinuses with transillumination, the diagnostic technique the otolaryngologist had used. It takes a special kind of X ray called a tomogram.

Now we were onto something! We felt the way Woodward and Bernstein must have felt when they first met Deep Throat. That doctor had incorrectly diagnosed June's problem and was treating her for the wrong condition. All June needed, we unholistically thought, was a doctor who knew what he was doing.

We decided to stop messing around and go for broke—a Beverly Hills doctor. A friend whose husband is a well-known internist recommended another otolaryngologist because that was the only kind of specialist we knew to ask for. After all, we reasoned, headaches are in the head and so are the areas in which otolaryngologists specialize.

June went to the Beverly Hills specialist with high hopes, but also with a slight touch of cynical deviousness. She didn't plan to tell him that she'd already been diagnosed or misdiagnosed as a victim of infected ethmoids.

The doctor took some X rays this time and came up

with a diagnosis of ethmoid sinuses, again. June's face and heart fell. It's the same old story and, she thought as she saw him take out his prescription pad, probably the same old antibiotic.

## A DRUG ON THE MARKET

This time the prescription was for two drugs: Stelazine and Polaramine.[1] After leaving the doctor's office, June raced to the library to find out what they were. She looked them up in the *Physician's Desk Reference*. The *PDR* tells everything a doctor (or patient) could want to know about any drug. Stelazine was a tranquilizer and Polaramine was an antihistamine. Since neither was an antibiotic, we knew the doctor wasn't treating June for an infection. Now we were making progress! With the correct diagnosis, a cure was surely on the way.

June was supposed to take the Stelazine in the morning and the Polaramine at night. But unfortunately a morning tranquilizer turned her brain into oatmeal and caused her to drift through her work day softly bouncing against book shelves. When it came to writing, she could hardly compose a coherent sentence. She took it upon herself to reverse the order, taking the Stelazine when she went to bed and the Polaramine when she got up. This seemed to work. The headaches stopped and she could function again as a librarian and writer.

The only cloud in all this blue sky appeared when June was having her teeth cleaned and happened to mention to the dentist that she'd just been cured of a terrible bout of headaches by a couple of wonder drugs. When he heard that one of them was Stelazine, he rolled his eyes and remarked that Stelazine was a *really* powerful tranquilizer. No matter, thought June, the headaches are gone and that's what counts.

However, it nibbled disturbingly at the back of her mind that she, who had always been wholeheartedly

[1]We frequently use brand names of drugs. For their generic names, see Appendix A.

antidrug, would have to go through life popping two a day. Probably not, she reassured herself. It's just a matter of time.

It was just a matter of time. But not the way she thought. A few weeks later June awoke with the headache again fastened to the bridge of her nose and her eyeballs. It radiated pain—the same pain as before or slightly worse.

"Surely it will go away. It's probably just some kind of farewell performance. I'll keep taking the pills." Despite the pills the headache lasted four days, let up for a couple of days, and then started again. A definite and distressing pattern was developing. Back to the Beverly Hills doctor, who prescribed a new drug, Etrafon, which is a combination tranquilizer and antidepressant.

Another slight remission and then headaches again. The eternal return for still another prescription, another tranquilizer called Bellergal. It contained phenobarbital, which June knew to be habit-forming. While she was getting this prescription filled, she complained to the pharmacist about how many different drugs she was having to take, drugs that were doing her no good and perhaps a great deal of harm.

"Cheer up," he said, "you only have about ninety more to try." He wasn't kidding.

Bellergal gave no lasting relief either. Finally disgusted with the drug scene and with herself for being a part of it, June discontinued use.

To try to get some respite from the pain, she started experimenting with natural remedies for sinus trouble and headaches. After reading all the wheat-germ-in-the-sky promises in Adelle Davis's *Let's Eat Right to Keep Fit* and *Let's Get Well*, she methodically worked her way through almost the entire vitamin and mineral cabinet: A, $B_1$, Niacin, $B_{12}$, C, E, calcium, pantothenic acid, zinc, iodine.

The advantage of vitamins and minerals over drugs

was that they produced no noticeable side effects—but no direct effects either. That is to say, June's headaches remained untouched by natural-healing hands.

We both felt the need now to understand more about sinus trouble and the headaches it was supposedly causing. With a combination of questions to the doctor and our own reading of medical books, we narrowed June's problem down to vasomotor rhinitis, which creates vacuum headaches. These headaches occur when blood vessels in the nasal passages swell and cut off the air to the sinus cavities. Knowing this, our puzzle now was to find out why the blood vessels were swelling and how to keep them from doing so. The doctors' dynamic drug duos hadn't worked, but what else was there?

## UP IN THE AIR

At this murky point in the mystery we were planning another European working vacation. Two days before departure June got the most horrendous headache of her career up to this time. She didn't want to go but, since it was too late to get a refund on the charter flight and since she figured she couldn't feel any worse in Europe, she went ahead with her plans.

When the plane had been off the ground for only ten minutes, a miracle occurred. June's headache cleared up. Totally. Was it the altitude? Was it just coincidence? We didn't know. And despite all the rigors and strains of travel she didn't have even a suspicion of a headache for the entire trip.

Two days after we returned to Los Angeles the headache was back. Several days on, a few days off. The same old pattern. With a kind of instinctive holism, we started trying to analyze the situation. Was it something other than her sinuses that was causing the problem? Was it something in Los Angeles or around her house?

We decided to experiment. The next time she was in the

throes of a headache, June threw a few things in the car and drove to Ojai, a resort community about 80 miles north of Los Angeles. In three hours the headache was gone and it stayed away all the while she was there.

Back in town, back came the headache. Now we were on to something.

June fled town with each headache. The results were always the same—an almost immediate alleviation of the pain. What, we asked ourselves, does Los Angeles have more of than any place else? The answer was not hard to find. It was all around, a sickly yellow-brown miasma. Smog. We started noticing the high-level, smog-alert pollution days and found that frequently they would trigger a headache. We also discovered that a change in the weather, especially a rise in the humidity before a rain, would break the headaches and give June a few days of relief.

Maybe if it's the Los Angeles air, we thought, she could get rid of the headaches with a straight shot of pure oxygen. Barbara, who suffers from altitude sickness (including headaches) on the first couple of days of a ski trip, owned a little handy-dandy oxygen kit. June tried breathing from that when she had a headache. No relief.

Well, how about an air purifier? If she put one of those in her bedroom, she could breathe clean air all night while she was asleep and all day while she was at home. If she had good air about half the time, that might be enough to keep the headaches away. June rented an air purifier from Abbey Rents and kept it running constantly for a month. Absolutely no improvement.

June made an appointment with her Beverly Hills otolaryngologist "just to talk." When she told him about our experiments and asked him if he thought it would do any good to move out of the Los Angeles area, he didn't talk equivocal medicalese: "If you lived somewhere like Lake Arrowhead, you'd never even know you had sinuses."

We figured he hadn't said anything about moving before because how do you tell a person to rip up roots and move to cure a headache? Most people won't or can't. And a move from Los Angeles wouldn't be easy for June, either. Obviously it would be a change that would turn her life inside out and upside down and into every other abnormal position. But what choice was there? In the year and a half since the headaches began, she was—at first slowly and then like a rock rolling down hill faster and faster—turning into what we had come to call a chronic headachoholic. She was no longer a person, just a container for pain. Something had to be done, so she did it. She sold her house and moved.

## DESERT CAMPAIGN

June's move was to the Mohave Desert community of Apple Valley, famous for its clear air and "champagne climate" as the real estate ads put it. It was a two-hour drive each way from June's work in the San Fernando Valley. In order to hold up under the stress and strain of the drive, she cut down to a three-fifths work assignment (with three-fifths salary), working only Mondays, Wednesdays, and Fridays.

For two years this plan worked—sort of. The headaches did diminish, but it wasn't the remarkable cure June had hoped for. Usually she was free from headaches in the winter months but when a heavy smog period hit Los Angeles, back they came and she'd often have to cut and run to the desert in the middle of the workday because she felt too terrible to function on the job.

It was a lonely and exhausting existence, but she held on. Then an ominous cloud began appearing on the desert horizon. On the days when the champagne climate popped its cork with the shrieking winds for which the area is famous, the sky began to turn that old familiar sickly yellow-brown color. The smog was blowing in from the metropolitan areas bringing with it headaches. Since the smog had followed her to the desert, June didn't know where to run.

## PUNCTURED HOPES

When she needed it most, June finally got a break. At the twenty-fifth anniversary celebration of the Valley College she found herself talking to one of the former presidents, who was a nonpracticing osteopath. Always on the alert for medical information, she brought up the subject of her headaches. He said he thought he knew of something that might help—acupuncture. He told her there was a new acupuncture institute right in the San Fernando Valley and that he'd had good reports on it.

It was such a great idea that we wondered why we hadn't thought of it ourselves. A TV program we had seen had shown how surgery could be performed and babies delivered using no anesthetic except for a few slender, painless needles stuck in strategic spots. Surely if acupuncture could stop that kind of pain, a headache wouldn't stand a chance.

June quickly called the institute and made the appointment for her initial interview with the M.D. who was in charge.

The office wait broke the record: two hours with one hour in a pseudo-Chinese room in the company of a large collection of dismal and damaged people of the sort you might find seeking a miracle cure at Lourdes and with another hour in one of the many treatment rooms.

When the weary-looking doctor finally arrived, June stated her problem: vasomotor rhinitis with vacuum headaches. She also mentioned all the drug flunkouts. The doctor seemed familiar with the problem. He said that 80 percent of those affected with that kind of headache got a three-year remission with around ten acupuncture treatments. June appreciated the honesty of the word "remission" rather than "cure." She was ripping to begin her three years of freedom from pain.

Not so fast. The doctor would only start the treatments when June was actually having a headache. (This happened to be one of the few days when she was having a respite. It was the first time she ever wished she had a headache.)

At the first onslaught of pain, June was to call in and she would be fitted into that day's schedule. (That doctor had quite a schedule. It ran from 9:00 A.M. to midnight!)

The headache clamped on. June called for her appointment. It was made for 8:00 P.M., but she wasn't taken into the treatment room until 9:30. The doctor appeared at 10:15. After telling her, "It's better not to look when I do this," he inserted fifty (she counted!) needles from the soles of her feet to the top of her head. All the stories you may have heard to the contrary, the acupuncture was a very painful process.

When the doctor finished, the nurse wired certain of the needles to an electric current and heated the rest of them with a burning stick of moxa (wormwood), which sent up a thick stream of pungent smoke. After the needles had been in for about half an hour, they were removed and so was $50 from June's bank account.

She staggered out of the office at 11:00 P.M., both bloody and bowed. Her head was still aching but by the next afternoon the headache was gone. Although it was still gone two days later, she had another treatment because she had been put on a four-treatment schedule. The next three sessions were all just as painful and debilitating as the first one, but *the acupuncture worked*! The headaches ended and though weeks passed, then months, they didn't return. June happily abandoned the desert and moved back to town.

Now that the mask of pain was lifted from her face, June looked wonderful, just like her old self. She began seeing friends again, now that she knew she wouldn't have to break dates because of a sudden onslaught of the headache. One Sunday she invited Barbara and the editor of our first three books over for brunch. The editor—as some editors are wont to do—usually smoked incessantly but restrained herself because she knew from past experience with June that cigarette smoke, just like smog, triggered her headaches.

Barbara assured her that it was OK to smoke now because "June's cured. She doesn't get headaches anymore." We had a wonderful time, a real celebration.

Two hours after the guests left, June had a headache. She wasn't terribly worried, though. After all, she hadn't had the magic ten treatments yet.

The next treatment released her from her headache for a while, a short while. Back for another treatment. And another. And another. It began to work out that the headaches came closer and closer together until she was getting them every two or three days just as before she started acupuncture.

When the basic ten treatments were over, the doctor thought June should continue to see if she could get another, longer remission. But the cost started becoming a consideration. Even more significantly, June began to feel she could no longer endure the stress and pain of going into the doctor's office for another session. When the pain of the treatment becomes almost as bad as the pain of the problem it's treating, there's a natural tendency to give up the treatment. June gave it up.

With the headaches back in full force, and always worse when the smog was heavy, June's only choice was to move again. As soon as the college semester ended, she rented an apartment in Laguna Beach, a perfect resort area with a perfect climate and as smog-free as you can get in Southern California.

It was an ideal summer for June. She had only one headache and that was because she went inland for lunch on a day when the smog hung hot and heavy.

In September when the college semester opened, June again opted to work Mondays, Wednesday, and Fridays, driving in and out of the city each day. The headaches returned following their regular pattern, usually beginning when she was at work.

## A SHOT IN THE DARK

Then one more hope for the headachoholic appeared on the horizon. We were giving a talk to an American Diabetes Association seminar. After the speech Barbara was talking to a diabetic woman and as usual the topic of June's chronic headaches came up.

This woman offered her theory that diabetics are particularly sensitive to allergies and, although most people picture allergy victims as coughing, sneezing, and blowing their noses, a headache is a very common allergy symptom. She, herself, had had chronic headaches for seven years until a doctor finally diagnosed them correctly as allergy symptoms. She had taken desensitization treatments and now rarely had headaches. She gave Barbara the name of the allergist who had cured her.

Although June had entered into her hostility-toward-doctors phase, she did consent to call for an appointment the next day. The fact that a headache came on right after the conference helped her to make the decision.

A lengthy history taking, another complete physical, and a battery of skin patch tests revealed that June had a mild allergy to olive and walnut trees; cattle, hog, horse, and cat dander; and household dust. The doctor was of the opinion that allergic rhinitis *might* (with about a 50 percent chance) be the cause of her headaches. To find out for sure she needed desensitization injections twice a week for at least six months. Regularly. No breaks in the pattern or she would have to start all over again.

June began the twice-a-week shots. Along with the first shot she was given a set of instructions for changing her lifestyle. Since one of her allergies was household dust, she was to remove as much of it as possible from her living quarters. Her mattress and pillows had to be covered with plastic cases. All throw rugs and every dust-catching bibelot had to be stored away. All furniture and carpeting and drapes had to be sprayed with Allergex ($5 a can). June was supposed to vacuum the entire apartment every other day wearing a dust mask much like the surgical masks the Japanese wear in order not to spread colds. And to top it all off, she was always to avoid sitting on up-holstered furniture. And never, *never* to keep company with a cow, horse, hog, or cat.

About every other shot of allergens gave June a headache. This delighted her because, she reasoned, if shots could bring on headaches, then the headaches must be caused by an allergic reaction. But her delight began to fade as the nurse kept dropping the strength of the dosage to try to keep the shots from causing headaches.

As time passed June not only made no progress, she went backward. After five months on the program her injections were at a lower level than when she began. She lost faith in the allergy theory and was ready to quit, but just to make sure she wasn't giving up too easily, she went back to the allergist for a reevaluation. He agreed that she wasn't getting anywhere. Allergies apparently weren't her problem. There was no point in going on.

Now even Barbara in her heart of hearts and head of heads began to think that what everyone always says about women's headaches might be true in June's case. She *could* be just whomping them up out of her neuroses. Maybe what she did need was a shrink. But it was no use trying to get her to one. She was even more negative on psychia-trists than she was getting to be on regular doctors. In fact, she always subscribed to Sam Goldwyn's philosophy: "Anyone who goes to a psychiatrist ought to have his head examined."

It was time to start another year at the college and there June was again without hope and with her head now socked in about 30 percent of the time with the pain of a headache. (She was even getting headaches in Laguna Beach now.) After four and a half years of pain, it got to be too much for her. She started talking about how she wasn't herself anymore (she wasn't), how she didn't like herself (well, frankly, she wasn't very likeable), and how she just might as well go into the garage and turn on the car for all the use she was to herself or anyone else.

This was scary talk. Barbara had read enough psychology to know that people who talk about suicide frequently go through with it. Since June had obviously given up, Barbara knew it was up to her to find a cure. Soon.

## HEAD MAN

In her quest for a cure Barbara started talking to the group on our campus that she referred to as the "headache underground." These were four women faculty members who were chronic headache sufferers. One of these sister headachoholics delivered the news that she had heard that a headache clinic had opened in Thousand Oaks, a resort-residential community north of Los Angeles.

Now that Barbara realized there were such things as headache clinics, she had a new line of attack. She called the UCLA Medical School to see whether they had one on the premises. They didn't but recommended Dr. Gunnar Heuser, a member of their teaching staff who in private practice specialized in treating headaches. His office was in Thousand Oaks. Now she had a double endorsement of her man.

It wasn't easy to get June to make the appointment, but Barbara finally badgered her into it and drove her to Thousand Oaks to make sure she got there.

Yes, there was an hour-long wait, but at least there was no one but us in the waiting room. This first visit was a full hour interview with Dr. Heuser, who had a soft German accent and looked like an Austrian ski instructor. He already knew a lot about June's medical history because she had sent him the records from all of her previous doctors. His first questions focused on the headaches. He asked her to rate her headache pain on a one-to-ten scale. Although she felt that no one had ever suffered more from headaches, she knew that such things as foot cramps and terminal cancer can be higher on the pain intensity scale, so she gave herself a conservative six.

Next he asked her how often she had headaches. On the advice of one of the members of the headache underground she had been keeping a headache diary during the weeks prior to the appointment. She was able to come right back with "30 percent of my waking hours."

When the doctor learned that she had been having chronic headaches for five years, he advanced his theory that when you have had headaches for a number of years, there is probably more than one contributing factor. And in the questions that followed, he was obviously checking out the many possible causes.

One question June remembers particularly was, "Have you ever had a whiplash or other injury to the neck or head?" More in fun than anything else June replied, "The only head injury I've ever had was when my brother socked me one when I was about eight. My jaw still cracks when I chew." Dr. Heuser seemed to consider this significant and carefully noted it on his clipboard.

The session ended with his description of a number of experiments that June was to perform at home in the two weeks before the next appointment. Among these were to follow a certain diet, to take prescribed high potency vitamins (C and B), and to perform such medically unorthodox tests as chewing bubblegum to see if heavy jaw work would bring on a headache and wearing a mood ring to check hand temperatures during headaches.

When the interview was finished, Dr. Heuser, knowing of Barbara's involvement in the case, came into the waiting room to talk with her. When she asked, only half kidding, whether he thought we were going to have to send June to the psychiatrist whose office was next door, he answered with a slow smile, "No, I don't think so quite yet. She has not by any means explored every possibility."

After we left June said, "That's the first doctor I've been to who gave me my money's worth." She especially appreciated the fact that he had worked with no preconceived notions. Never did he mention vasomotor rhinitis, migraine headaches, or any other headache label. Instead, he was exploring many possibilities simultaneously and—what June appreciated most—was allowing her to participate in the exploration. She wasn't just passively being stuck or injected with needles or doped with drugs. Oh, yes, that was the best part of all. The doctor confessed to June, "I'm not much of a drug man," and didn't prescribe any for June. And a good thing, too. June says in retrospect, "I wouldn't have taken them if he had."

It was, in short, a perfect meeting of holistic minds.

On her second appointment June didn't have much to report. The headaches were still appearing in their usual 30 percent pattern. The diet changes didn't seem to make any difference. None of the experiments had yielded significant results.

For the physical examination scheduled for this visit, Dr. Heuser took a different approach than June had experienced in all her many other physicals. This exam was primarily a neurological and muscular one—scratching the bottom of the foot to see how the toes curled, hitting the knee with a little hammer to check the reflexes, looking for asymmetry in the legs, back, and posture, and checking for tight and tender areas in various muscle groups.

There was also a temporomandibular joint check. This is the joint on each side of the jaw that allows you to open and close your mouth and move your chin from side to side. This is the joint that cracked when June chewed. If this joint is out of alignment or damaged, it can cause chronic headaches that masquerade as migraines. Dr. Heuser's check involved pressing in front of her ears below the temples while she opened and closed her mouth to see if there was any soreness. Yes, there was. Dr. Heuser thought TMJ (as temporomandibular joint is often abbreviated) might be partially responsible for June's headaches. For a definite diagnosis he recommended that she see either of the two Los Angeles dentists, Dr. Victor Mintz and Dr. Arnold Greene, who specialized in treating the condition.

Dr. Heuser made a point of assuring June that, based on the tests he had run plus her previous CAT scan (computerized axial tomography scan, a special kind of brain X ray), she had "no cerebral pathology for tumor." That is medicalese for "Relax, you don't have a brain tumor." We found out later that tumors are the headache sufferer's greatest fear, although they're rarely the cause of chronic headaches.

June was instructed to come in the next day she had a headache so that Dr. Heuser could try to diagnose what type or types she had. She was assigned a few more experiments to perform. And that was that. Nary a lab test, blood test, X ray, blood pressure, pulse, weighing, none of the routine that had so irritated June.

By this time June had gone through a complete attitude reversal. She had become a cooperative and enthusiastic patient, a holistic participant in her cure. She even made an immediate appointment with one of the dentists that Dr. Heuser had recommended. Having nothing else to go by, she chose Dr. Arnold Greene because he was nearby in the San Fernando Valley.

## JAWS

After Dr. Greene ran a quick series of TMJ tests on June, he announced that he was positive that he could cure her headaches. He told her she was a textbook TMJ syndrome case. On the old one-to-ten scale she was a solid eight because she had the problem on only one side. Otherwise, she'd have broken the bank. June thought to herself, I've heard this song before. It's another invitation to membership in the cure-of-the-month club.

Apparently reading the skepticism on her face, Dr. Greene elaborated. What he had to do was construct a dental plane to correct her bite. This would cost $500 and, since neither medical nor dental insurance recognized this treatment, June had to pay the entire cost.

Seeing June draw back at the price, he continued, "Usually I require patients to pay the entire amount in advance, but you can pay for the work as it's done and you begin to notice the results. And I'm certain you *will* notice results."

Almost as if another person were talking, she heard herself say, "When can we begin?"

The bite plane was ready on her next visit. It looked something like a retainer and fit over the lower four rear teeth on each side. It built up the molars to the proper height, or at least a step in that direction. Dr. Greene warned June to keep it in her mouth at all times. He especially wanted her to wear it at night, because that's when the major clenching and bruxing (grinding) take place, bringing on TMJ headaches. He assured June that most of his patients' headaches cleared up immediately after they got their plane. She left his office with hopes as high as the new level of her molars.

After scheduling her next appointment for two weeks later, June went to Laguna Beach for Christmas vacation. After two days there, she received a negative Christmas present—a headache, the worst one she'd ever experienced. It seems that every headache June has is spotlighted as *the* worst, but truly this was it. The proof is that Ms. Antidrug herself staggered to the medicine cabinet, sorted among her vast collection of zonkers, and swallowed a Nembutal.

After June had suffered for two days a strange and miraculous thing happened. The phone rang. It was Dr. Greene inquiring how she was getting along. (He really cared!)

After hearing her vivid agony report, he told her to take out the plane and leave it out until her next appointment.

A few hours after June had removed the plane, the headache departed and stayed away for the rest of the vacation.

When June reported to Dr. Greene, he discovered that the plane was too high and said that was what had brought on her stupendous headache.

A likely story, she thought.

He adjusted the plane and cautioned her to come in immediately if she felt a headache coming on.

For the next three weeks Dr. Greene made plane adjustments whenever June began to experience the slightest twinge of a headache or even the slightest strange feeling in the head. She didn't get any more devastating headaches, but she still had about the usual number of average ones plus waves of strange, unpleasant feelings in the head.

While June was still in this state of confusion as to whether the plane was doing harm or good or nothing at all, the moment of financial truth arrived. It was payment time. June had to decide whether to go on with the treatment and commit herself to the full $500 or not.

When she went to her next appointment with Dr. Greene, she *still* hadn't made up her mind. Would she or wouldn't she?

It turned out that she would. Not, as she explained later, because she had any certainty that the TMJ syndrome was the question or the plane the answer, but because "I couldn't drop out on a man who had worked so hard to help me. Actually, he'd already earned the $500 on his time alone."

Then the headaches ended. Just like that—not with a

bang, not with a whimper, not with anything. They just silently stole away and didn't come back. Oh, yes, they did give one last command performance when Dr. Greene insisted that June take out the plane to eliminate coincidence and to prove beyond any doubt that the plane was what had solved her problem.

June was reluctant but she complied. It took two nights and three days for her to get a headache. The pain then lasted for four nights and four days. That was all the proof she needed and all the experimenting she was ever willing to do again. In fact, she promptly decided to make the cure permanent by investing $4,200 in permanent crowns for her lower back teeth.

The date of that last headache was March 5, 1976, and unless you see an erratum note inserted into the front of this book, June's headaches have been permanently arrested.

Case closed.


## THE CLOUDY SOLUTION

Agatha Christie's editor would never have let her get away with writing a mystery that had an ending as shrouded in unanswered questions as June's headache mystery story. You shouldn't let us get away with it either, not if you want to use June's detective story as a paradigm for solving your own headache mystery. We obviously haven't given you the whole solution yet. There are still many unanswered questions and many red herrings left to fry.

Why did June's headaches suddenly start after the bout with the flu? Why did two reputable physicians diagnose the condition as vasomotor rhinitis? Why did the headaches seem to come on during periods of high smog and in the presence of cigarette smoke? Why did they diminish before a rainstorm? Why did they go away as soon as June left the ground in an airplane? Why did acupuncture work for a while and then fail? Why did the allergy shots bring on a headache? Why did June never have a headache during a vacation away from home and work?

For these many whys we have no definite becauses, but we do have a theory.

## THE DAM THEORY: WATER OVER THE BRIDGE

The key to June's headache mystery lies in Dr. Heuser's theory that when you have had the headaches for a number of years, there is probably more than one contributing factor. The English author of *Do Something About That Migraine*, Dr. K. M. Hays, says in his quaint British way that some headache sufferers "have learned that they must avoid certain things in life that can act as triggers. It is usual for several of these factors to be acting together to precipitate a paroxism."

Based on these statements and on our own observations of June's headaches, we have evolved our own dam theory for those damn headaches. Imagine a dam, behind which there is a reservoir. Rain, hail, sleet, snow, and various runoffs from the mountains all cause the water level behind the dam to rise. When too many of these factors combine, the water spills over the top of the dam, causing a devastating flood in the valley below.

Headaches work in a similar way. Elements such as stress, fatigue, air pollution, weather changes, allergies, diseases and infections, certain foods and drinks, and various other psychological and physiological factors can combine to spill over into a devastating headache.

The way we analyze June's problem is that the TMJ syndrome always kept the water behind her headache dam at about the half-way point. June's damaged ethmoids raised it another few feet. The physical and emotional stresses of diabetes pushed the level a little higher while her slight allergies caused another rise. The water rose still higher because of the daily pressures of work and life. Then came weather changes and cigarette smoke and air pollution, and the whole collection spilled over into a headache. The smog frequently was the last drop that made the water spill over the dam, creating the false impression that it was the primary factor causing the headaches.

There is still another headache-augmenting possibility. When under stress, June would clamp her misaligned jaw and grind her teeth, bringing on a TMJ headache. Indeed, Daniel E. Lupton, writing about TMJ in the *American Dental Association Journal*, said, "Without nervous tension ... such dysfunction would not occur even though the mechanical and physiological factors may be present." When June saw smog or cigarette smoke, she would often start to fret and fear a headache, clamp and grind, and promptly get one. The fact that she never got a headache while on vacation is explained by the fact that she was away from life's stresses and had nothing to clamp and grind about.

Now that the TMJ problem is resolved the water behind June's headache dam starts at zero instead of the half-way point. Consequently, she can accommodate most of the other headache-inducing elements (many of which cannot be avoided) without a spill.

On the basis of this dam theory it is almost certain that you're going to be looking for more than one culprit in your headache detective work. Your job — with our help — will be to identify every one of the malfeasants no matter what disguises they may wear, and to arrest them with the holistic techniques we are going to reveal to you.

# 3

## YOUR MYSTERY HEADACHE

Now it is time for you to start your own holistic detective work, to solve your own headache mystery. How are you going to approach it? We hope with that good old Scotland Yard combination of brains, logic, and perseverance plus a wide-open mind. You'll also need to lay in a large supply of that vital medication, tincture of patience. Nothing is going to happen overnight. It took a while for you to get yourself into your mystery and it's going to take a while for you to get yourself out of it. We don't believe, however, it will take you nearly as long as it took June, because you'll have the benefit of her experiences and our research in both the conventional and the holistic approaches to health.

In the beginning the most important thing for you to do is to acknowledge the fact that you have a mystery by calling your headache what it is: an *idiopathic* headache. Idiopathic, despite the sound of it, has nothing to do with low-level intelligence. It just means the cause of the problem is unknown.

We've learned from June's experience that slapping a label on a headache early on in the search wastes a great deal of time. June used up three years and endured what seemed to be centuries of pain wearing the label of vasomotor rhinitis. Another year went down the drain bearing the banner of allergic rhinitis. She even was briefly marked migraine.

Migraine is the worst of all possible headache labels to pin on yourself or have pinned on you by a doctor. Just as "the butler did it" is the cliché of mystery stories, migraine is the cliché of chronic headache diagnosis. We have read in medical literature and heard at medical conferences on headaches about the percentage of chronic headaches that are actually classic migraines. Although the exact numbers vary depending on which doctor is reporting, the figures are always very low—between 7 percent and 10 percent. Yet virtually every one of the estimated 38 million American women headache sufferers has been branded "migraine sufferer" by her doctors and herself. Migraine usually is used as a synonym for any recurring excruciating headache that no one knows how to cure.

Not only that, but even bona fide migraine sufferers almost always experience muscular tension headaches in between their migraine bouts. Indeed, one theory has it that muscular tension headaches can trigger migraines and, therefore, if you could stop *them*, perhaps the migraine would be mostly dammed up as well.

We've also learned from experience that it's not just doctors who have the headache misnomer and mistreatment habit. In her desperation to find the cause and cure, the headache sufferer will latch on to anyone else's cause and cure and try to make it her own. That's what June did with the woman who had the allergy headaches. After we talked with her, we tore off to the University of California at Irvine Medical School library and read everything we could find on the subject of allergies. It turned out that every word we read on allergy-induced headaches rang true. June appeared to be a textbook allergic rhinitis case. This trap of finding yourself in any symptom complex you read about is known as the medical student syndrome. June fell headlong into it. Don't you.

If you try to fit your headaches into someone else's mold, you'll only set yourself back. You could spend months or years going to the wrong doctor for the wrong treatment. "But," you may protest, "if it's the wrong treatment, the doctor won't give it to me, will he?" He very well might, and not out of any unethical profit-making motive, either. Although there are some doctors who can't stand to turn away potential fees and others whose egos won't allow them to admit ignorance or defeat on any medical problem, these are the exception.

More often a doctor may believe, in good faith, that what ails you is in his area of expertise and that he *can* help. As Dr. Greene once said to June, "Surgeons will cut." And, we might add, allergists will give desensitization shots, otolaryngologists will give you the hose-in-the-nose and drugs, acupuncturists will stick in needles, psychiatrists will do whatever it is they do, and internists will keep referring you to other specialists when you continually appear in their offices bleating, "Doctor, you've got to do *something*. I can't stand the pain." And most of these doctors will be treating you with the best of intentions.

Not only is it unlikely that these treatments will help your headaches, but their side effects may make things worse. You may, in fact, wind up with an *iatrogenic* illness, which means a doctor- or treatment-induced illness, such as June's allergy-shot headaches.

Of course, it is possible that you could accidentally stumble upon the cause and cure of your headaches in this secondhand way. Accidents do happen and even Scotland Yard must occasionally solve a crime by happenstance but, in headache detection, a logical, careful, step-by-step approach is almost always the best and certainly the shortest route to a cure.

## VASCULAR OR MUSCULAR?

Now we've taken away the one clue you thought you had—a headache label—but we aren't going to leave you suspended there in midache with no hint whatsoever on how to classify your headache. The truth is that headaches can be divided into two general types, vascular and muscular. Knowing which type you predominantly have is useful in deciding which of the following tests and experiments are more significant in your case and which temporary relief measures in Chapter 5 will work best for you. (Though we must warn you that you can have one kind of headache at one time and the other at another time or even both at the same time.)

In vascular headaches there are changes in the blood vessels in the head that alter the amount of blood flowing there. Usually it's a matter of the dilation of the blood vessels, which causes pressure on the nerves. Muscular headaches, on the other hand, develop when muscles contract as a result of strained body positions, infections, accidents, emotional tension, or allergic reaction. Muscular headaches vastly outnumber vascular ones. Janet Travell, who gave John F. Kennedy the wonderfully holistic back-pain remedy of sitting in a rocking chair, believes that 90 percent of headaches are of musculoskeletal origin. She calls them "mechanical" headaches.

We have a simple and entertaining way for you to find out whether your headaches are primarily vascular or muscular. This is one of the unorthodox diagnostic aids Dr. Heuser used to solve June's headache mystery. Get yourself a mood ring. These are the rings with a stone that changes color, supposedly as your mood changes. They say that the stone is a bright blue when you're happy and black when you're depressed. In reality the stone is not affected by your mood but by the temperature of your hands. When your hands are warm, the stone is the "happy" color. When they're cold, the stone turns to the "depressed" shade.

If you wear a mood ring all the time and find it invariably turns black when you have a headache, that's an indication your headaches are at least partially vascular. When June wore the mood ring the stone did vary in color from time to time, but was not necessarily black when she had a headache. In other words, according to the ring, her headaches were not vascular. The mood ring's diagnosis later proved to be correct since the TMJ problem is a muscular one.

A second simple and entertaining way for you to check yourself out, if you're not a teetotaler or a minor or an alcoholic, is the alcohol test. If you find that having a couple of drinks makes your headache better, it's probably muscular. If alcohol makes your headache worse, it's probably vascular. Alcohol, in case you didn't realize it, is an effective muscle relaxant. In fact, one dentist told us it's the only effective muscle-relaxing drug there is, but he can't prescribe it because of its harmful side effects on the kidneys and liver and its addictiveness.

Another test—this one for muscular headaches only—is to try touching your toes while keeping your knees straight. If you can only get down a little beyond your knees, this indicates that your muscles are stiff and tense, making you a good candidate for muscular headaches. Also, tilt your head back and gaze at the ceiling. If this makes you dizzy it could mean tight neck muscles, which can cause headaches.

## CRIME DETECTION

We know there is nothing that doctors warn against more than self-diagnosis and self-treatment. But when it comes to headache mysteries, the solution depends in part on the results of investigations only you can perform. The investigations we're going to tell you about now fall into this category.

There are no experiments here that could cause you

any harm unless, as you carry them out, you delay seeking medical treatment while a tumor crowds into your brain cells. However, brain tumor is a very uncommon cause of headaches. (Only one headache patient in 1,600 had a tumor in one British study.) If you are one of the few chronic sufferers who has never been to a doctor for headache diagnosis, before going any further you should at least have an M. D. check you for what they call "cerebral pathology for tumor." This is done with a CAT scan (computerized axial tomography scan), which shows normal and abnormal intracranial structures. This X-ray technique can definitely rule out brain tumor as a cause of your headache.

From the start you should be aware that you will have to conduct several of these experiments at the same time. Remember the Great Truth of the dam theory: If you have had chronic headaches over a period of time, they most likely have more than one contributing factor. And it follows that the more causes, the more experiments you must perform if you are to solve your mystery or to provide the information a doctor will need to help you solve it.

## SEVEN SWORDS

We heard a psychologist vividly and accurately describe chronic headaches as the "disease of the seven swords." Think of a woman with seven swords sticking into her, as if a magician had pierced her as part of his act. Except in this case it's no trick. The swords are really sticking into the woman and she's in extreme pain. Seeking a release from her suffering, she goes to a doctor who looks her over and says, "Ah, ha! It's *this* sword that's causing your problem." He pulls out that sword. "Is the pain gone?" "No, it isn't." "Well, then, it mustn't be that sword after all." He sighs and sticks the sword back in.

The woman goes to another doctor, who says, "I think it's *this* sword." He pulls out a different sword, but still the pain persists. Back in goes that sword. On she goes to another doctor where the same thing happens again. The woman is never free from pain, because only one sword at a time is ever removed.

It is important, therefore, that you or your doctor simultaneously pull as many swords—remove as many potential headache causes—as possible from your life by availing yourself of as many experiments mentioned in this book as you can at one time. You should also conduct the experiments over a long enough period of time—usually several weeks—to show valid results. In order to avoid having to live with these restrictions forever, what you can do after the headaches stop or diminish is to gradually put back the swords *one at a time* until you find the basic ones that are truly causing *your* headaches.

We must emphasize the importance of keeping accurate records of the results of these experiments. In the next chapter we'll show you how to do this in a special headache diary.

You can see that this process of crime detection is not going to be easy and it's not going to be quick. But if chronic headaches were easily and quickly cured, yours would be gone by now, wouldn't they?

## ALLERGY SWORDS

### What You Eat

There's probably no food or drink to which someone isn't allergic. June happens to be allergic to cucumbers, Barbara to mussels. An allergy to one food often means that a person will be allergic to related foods as well. But certain foods are more notorious offenders than others in triggering headaches. For example, in 1904 the English physician Alexander Haig observed that severe migraine could be reduced by a diet that was low in meat and salt.

We always recall the case of one chronic headache patient, who had the habit of finishing off her breakfast every morning with a couple of M and M's (those little chocolate-centered candies that melt in your mouth, not in your hands). Unfortunately, in her case they also melted into a headache, since she turned out to be allergic to chocolate, which is at the very top of the list of headache-causing food allergies.

Sometimes the headache doesn't seem to be related to food or drink but is. For example, one man had what he called a "laughing headache"—it literally only hurt when he laughed. It took a long time before he and his doctor deduced that the patient only laughed when he drank beer. The headache was really a beer-allergy headache. It wasn't an alcohol-induced headache because he didn't get it when he drank whiskey—and he didn't for some reason laugh when he drank whiskey either. We will discuss headaches related to alcohol and alcoholic beverages later.

In interviews with doctors and in library research we have heard and read over and over again that food allergies are underrated as a cause of headaches. Then again, just to show you how few certainties there are in the world of headache treatment, a 1978 study headed by Dr. Seymour Diamond, director of the Diamond Headache Clinic in Chicago, came up with the information that diet has no connection with headaches. This is the kind of confusion that makes a person allergic to scientific information.

It is our point of view that we sufferers can afford to leave no stone—or bone—unturned. Therefore, we think the best decision would be to go along with the majority opinion and check out food triggers, as they're referred to in the allergy trade, with the greatest of dedication. And dedication *is* the word, because it's a job you have to do by yourself in true holistic fashion, except in rare instances.

Food tests are conducted in two ways: (1) total dietary restriction and (2) overload. Using the first method, you try to eliminate the headache by avoiding the offending food, and in the second you try to bring the headache on by saturating yourself with the food. The best system is to check food out using both methods. You start with the elimination of typically offensive foods for a two-week period and follow this by an overload.

Let's say you practice total dietary restriction of chocolate, eggs, milk, peanuts, and fish. During the two weeks of restriction you find your headaches are less frequent or intense than usual. So you ask yourself which of these foods you missed the most. What you missed the most is the most likely culprit. Then have an overload day for that food. If milk, for instance, was what you missed most, you'd have a "milk day" on which you drank plenty of milk and ate only foods that are basically "safe" or nonallergenic. (See the Safe Foods List, Appendix B.) If you get a terrific headache, then milk could be one of the contributing factors that is making you spill over your dam into headache pain. If you don't get a headache, milk is probably safe for you. Next, you'd have a "chocolate day," and then a "fish day," until you'd practiced overload with the entire list to see if you could create a headache with any of the foods being tested.

**The Big Seven.** We're going to list for you the seven foods that have the best established reputations as headache producers. To come up with this list we checked food lists in five of the currently most popular headache books (Brainard, Diamond, Friedman, Hass, and Speer) plus some lists we picked up from lectures by other doctors. Unfortunately, almost every doctor who has ever written a headache book seems to have come up with his own favorite list of what he would classify as the ten-most-wanted criminals of food-related headaches.

By tabulating them according to first place, second place, and so forth, we compiled a ranking of those foods that were the highest vote getters in the headache-causes election.

Here's our list of the "big seven." These are the foods you should deal with first in your two-week elimination tests.

1. & 2. Milk, Chocolate
3. Eggs
4. Wheat
5. Peanuts
6. Citrus fruit (including tomatoes)
7. Pork

Other foods among the headache-causing candidates included peas, all fresh fruits, all nuts, onions, spices and spicy food, legumes, shellfish, fish, and chicken.

A single one of these suspicious characters can be the major cause of someone's chronic headaches. The "peanut butter headache" is a classic example. Sometimes, however, the connection between the food and the headache is not all that obvious. We're thinking of the "doughnut headache." This is not caused by doughnuts but by the lard in which the doughnuts are cooked. Lard is pork fat and it's the allergy to pork that produces the headache. And then there's the "pizza headache," in which the headache is traceable to one simple ingredient of pizza, the tomatoes. So you see that in checking out the "big seven" you must analyze the composition of each food or food concoction you eat and not let yourself be tricked by some clever criminal in disguise.

**Vivonex.** For those of you who would like a shortcut food allergy test, there is a liquid diet called Vivonex that can be used as an overall "safe food" and that physicians can prescribe for you.

Vivonex is a synthetic balanced diet formula in powder form (made by Eaton Laboratories of Norwich, New York) that is sold in packages of 300 calories each. The powder comes unflavored or in vanilla, beef broth, grape, and in some flavors that can cause allergy headaches (chocolate and strawberry) and thus have to be avoided. The most palatable way to use Vivonex is to mix the unflavored variety with apple juice. And it's best to sip it all day long; in large doses it can give you diarrhea.

If you live on Vivonex for five to ten days and your headaches continue then you can rule out food allergy as a contributing factor in your case. If your headaches diminish or stop entirely while you're on Vivonex, then food may be a factor, and you then have to find out which foods are the headache producers by using the restriction-and-overload method.

One warning about launching into a Vivonex test. A basic human food satisfaction need is met by chewing. Many people find that, because this need isn't met with a liquid diet, they can't stick to it for the required period of time.

### What You Breathe

Allergy headaches can be brought on by what you breathe as well as by what you eat. You may have friends who sneeze or get tearing eyes and running noses in the spring when pollens are in the air or know someone who is allergic to cigarette smoke. But that's just a whiff of the possibilities. Individuals can be allergic to almost any flower, plant, tree, grass, mold, or fungus; to household dust, fur, and feathers; to gases, petroleum products, cosmetics, cleaning products, paint and paint products; and even to household odors like mothballs, newspapers, and frying oils.

We have an old friend who for several years was the victim of "marigold headaches" until her doctor diagnosed the source properly. Another woman had chronic headaches because she was allergic to the perfume worn by another woman in her office. (We wonder how you solve this one diplomatically.)

The trick here is to find out which airborne allergens (allergy inducers), if any, are contributing to your headaches. Simply becoming aware and suspicious of what you breathe may give you a lead, especially if you jot down your observations in your headache diary (see Chapter 4). Then you have to check out your clues by avoiding marigolds or perfume or whatever. You can also go to an allergist for skin scratch tests, as June did. And, finally, you can try the following home allergy testing method.

## Skin-Contact Home Allergy Testing

The world is so full of a number of things—foods and substances—to which you could be allergic that it's very difficult to pin down what might be causing an allergic reaction that manifests itself in headaches. You can't have skin tests for *everything*. There are just too many possibilities. Besides, skin tests are notoriously inaccurate in testing for food allergies.

If there are certain foods or substances with which you are in daily contact and that you suspect might be culprits in your headache crime, there is another way to find a clue that may pin the rap on them: skin-contact home allergy testing. Barbara heard about it from a chiropractor, Dr. Louise M. Laugen, who described both the technique and its rationale in a lecture at Valley College.

Several years ago another chiropractor, Dr. Riddler, ascertained that substances to which you are allergic cause muscle weakness. When he was performing muscle tests on a patient in his office in his home, Dr. Riddler discovered that the muscle he was working on suddenly lost strength. He couldn't figure out why. Then he noticed the family cat strolling out from under the examining table. The patient noticed the cat, too. "Better get that cat out of here," he said, "I'm allergic to them."

This incident set Dr. Riddler to thinking that there could be a physiological connection between allergies and loss of muscle strength, so he began experimenting. Based on his research he developed a new technique for allergy testing.

Dr. Riddler's technique is as follows. You will need another person to help you with the testing. For greatest accuracy wear very few clothes. Ideally, you should be nude. After all, you might be allergic to something you are wearing, and the resultant muscle weakness could invalidate the test results. Also remove all jewelry, since metals and precious stones can interfere with test reactions.

You can perform the test with virtually any muscle, but the easiest one to use is in the arm. When you're being tested, hold your arm straight out in front of you parallel to the ground, palm down. The person testing you then places one hand on your shoulder and the other on your arm just below the elbow and tries to push your arm down, while you try to keep it in the parallel-to-the-ground position. Usually it's fairly difficult for the tester to push your arm down when you're offering resistance.

Next, hold the suspected substance in the hand of the arm that is being tested. It's best to have the substance directly touching your hand but, if it's something that must be in a container, then the container should be composed of inorganic material such as plastic (it should *not* be made of glass, wood, or paper). When food is being tested, it can be either held in the hand or placed under the tongue.

Then test the muscle in exactly the same way as before with the tester applying the same amount of force. If you are allergic to the substance, your arm should go down very easily. It will seem as if your arm has lost all its strength.

Dr. Laugen pointed out that the advantage of this test, besides the fact that it's free and you can do it at home, is that you can test the things you actually eat, use, and are in daily contact with—the brand of peanut butter you buy, the detergent you use, the hair from your own cat or dog, and your own household dust. She believes this is a much more valid test than one using a standardized laboratory allergy test version of cat hair, household dust, etc.

Admittedly, this test smacks of that old black magic, so Barbara was somewhat skeptical. After Dr. Laugen demonstrated her test, Barbara walked to the library and pulled a few leaves from a handy olive tree. June, as you may recall, was diagnosed via the skin scratch test as having an allergy to olive trees. Without giving June any idea of what she was up to, Barbara conducted the test and, even though June had all her clothes and jewelry on, the test worked perfectly.

Since we didn't want to think of this test as being something occult, we tried to find a scientific basis for it. Dr. David Bresler, Ph.D., of the UCLA Pain Control Unit, told us that the technique works because people have sensory receptors all over their bodies including a number in their hands and under their tongues. These receptors can pick up allergens from offending substances and transmit them to the muscle, causing an almost instantaneous allergic weakening reaction.

Even more evidence of the validity of this test came from a psychiatrist who grinds up a suspect food and mixes it with distilled water. Only two drops of this mixture placed under the patient's tongue can produce startling allergic reactions—some psychological as well as physical.

These tests are certainly worth a try and, if you do find foods or substances that cause a muscle-weakening reaction, you can avoid them to see if your headaches decrease. Later on for a sure and certain diagnosis you can have an allergist test you with a conventional skin test.

A final allergy test that we suggest is to examine your parents. Heredity is very significant in allergies. If you have one parent with an allergy, you have a 40 percent chance of having one; if both parents have allergies, your chances can rise to as high as 80 percent.

## POSTURAL SWORDS

### Muscles: The Unlucky Seven

The number seven—seven swords, "big seven" foods—seems to be the key digit in headache crime detection. This time it's the seven muscles that contain pain trigger points to the head. These are shown in Fig. 1. By constantly holding any one of these muscles in a shortened or tightened position you can bring on chronic headaches. Let's go over some postural habits that create this very situation in order for you to check your own habits against them.

1. *Do you regularly hold your chin forward?* In this category we can put "bifocal headaches," headaches caused by sticking your chin forward to peer better through the reading portion of your glasses. June suspects this was a contributing factor in her headaches.

Also, some automobile commuters hold their chins forward as they drive the freeway for hours each day. Sometimes this can be corrected by moving the seat forward or by sitting on a pillow.

2. *Are you a frequent telephone user and, if so, how do you hold the phone?* One executive talked on the telephone most of his working day and had the habit of holding the telephone receiver between his left ear and his left shoulder. He developed a chronic headache on the left side of his head. His problem was solved by purchasing a telephone microphone, putting it directly in front of him, and holding his head straight while he worked.

3. *Do you always sleep on your stomach?* If so, your head is turned to one side and one muscle is shortened. This stiffens the muscle to an extreme, especially if you sleep a regular eight hours nightly. The solution is to train yourself to sleep on your side or on your back.

4. *Do you visit a beauty parlor for a once-a-week shampoo and set?* If so, it just might be that your headaches are related to this activity. One doctor's patient went to the beauty parlor every Saturday. Every Monday she developed a headache.

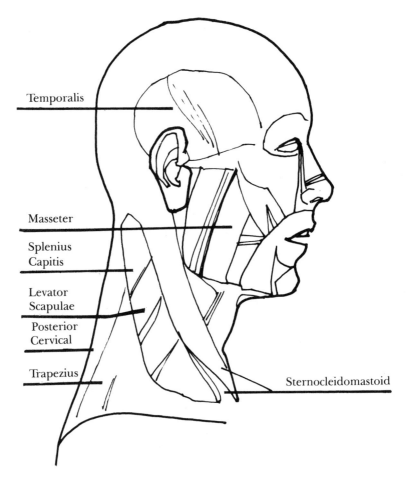

Temporalis

Masseter

Splenius
Capitis

Levator
Scapulae

Posterior
Cervical

Trapezius

Sternocleidomastoid

Figure 1

It turned out that her headaches were caused by having her head slung back over the basin—a very unnatural position—for shampooing. The cause was not easily identified, because there was a forty-eight-hour delay between the cause and effect. This delayed reaction often occurs with headache pain.

The trigger point for the "beauty parlor headache" is in the soft tissue at the base of the skull. When the muscles in this area are shortened by bending the head back, a pain can be referred to the area above your eyes or on top of your head. So here's a summation of the clues in this case: beauty parlor shampoo, headache follows a day or two afterwards, pain is over eyes and at top of head. The solution is simply to wash your hair at home before going to the beauty parlor or to ask your beautician to shampoo your hair in a forward bending position.

5. *Do you have an office job that requires typing most of the day?* You may lock yourself for too many hours at a time into a posture that eventually results in a muscle-contraction headache. For years June typed with her manuscript copy placed flat at the left side of the typewriter. Her head was always turned to the left and the left sternocleidomastoid muscle was held in a shortened position because her head was not only twisted in that direction but bent down to keep her eyes on the copy. The muscle was constantly tight and sore.

Since we've learned so much about muscles as a cause of pain, June has purchased a standing copy holder to which she attaches the sheets she's typing from. Now her neck is not so twisted to the left and her head is generally level. The result is a decrease of soreness in this muscle and a potential headache factor eliminated.

6. *Do you frequently lift heavy pots and pans?* Dr. David Rubin, a muscle rehabilitation expert at UCLA, mentioned in a lecture that women with headaches—all women, in fact—should avoid lifting heavy pots, such as cast iron, from lower shelves or hoisting them down from

higher shelves without a footstool. Straining muscles can change muscle tissue, even irreversibly. Then these changed areas develop trigger points that send pain to specific areas of the head. Oddly enough, just as in the "beauty parlor headache" the pain you feel can be located a long distance away from the muscle you've damaged.

7. *Do you have a car with manual transmission?* Operating the clutch pedal and shifting gears cause stress in several of the seven muscles that contain pain trigger points to the head. If you're spending a lot of time in heavy stop-and-go traffic, you might try not driving your car for a week unless, of course, you love your car more than you hate your headaches.

**Muscling Out: Relief.** If you find yourself regularly involved in one of the above muscle-shortening situations or some unique one of your own not mentioned here (these are only examples, after all), the first thing to do is to cease and desist.

You can also treat the offended-offending muscle that is contributing to your headache with heat or cold. People always seem to think of treating sore muscles with a heating pad or hot bath, but sometimes cold, which relaxes muscles so that they can be stretched, works better than heat, which causes swelling.

The cold treatment can be an ice pack or a spray. One spray, Fluori-Methane, requires a prescription, but another called Cramer Cold Spray does not. If you can't find the latter locally, it can be ordered from Starting Line Sports, P.O. Box 8, Mountain View, CA 94042. (Ask them for their *Complete Runner's Catalog* for details on their ordering procedure.)

Some muscle-tension headache sufferers have been helped by sleeping on a cylindrical cervical pillow. It supports the neck and upper shoulders while allowing the head to drop back and relax. The one we've heard the best reports on is called the Wal-Pil-O. If you can't find one of these at your local medical supply store you can write to Rolake Co., P.O. Box 24DD3, Los Angeles, CA 90024.

## Them Bones

Skeletal imbalances can also create headache pain. One clue we offer is an uneven wearing down of the heels of your shoes. This may indicate that one leg is shorter than the other. If so, your body's misalignment could be mostly responsible for you head pain.

Another test you might make to see if one leg is shorter than the other is to stand with your legs together and ask a friend to check and see if the creases in back of your knees are on the same level. If not, it's definitely something to mention to your doctor. We urge you to make this check because Dr. Joan Ullyot of the Institute for Health Research in San Francisco says that, according to some surveys, two thirds of all Americans have one leg shorter than the other.

One podiatrist had a young headache sufferer referred to him by an internist. On examination the podiatrist found that one of the patient's legs was shorter than the other and noticed that one of her arches was flattening out. He made orthotics for the young woman. These are plastic inserts that go into the shoe and control the motion of the feet, restricting the overcompensating motion she was making because of her shorter leg. Her headaches cleared up almost immediately.

**Chiropractic advice.** Many physicians admit that some of their muscle-tension headache patients have been helped by chiropractors. (Some physicians go to chiropractors themselves for pain relief.) A group of physicians has even formed an organization—The Society for Manipulative Medicine—to study this treatment.

When June developed a tightness and pain in her neck and shoulder muscles because of readjustments made on her bite plane after she started wearing it, she had several treatments from Dr. Gerald Pearlman, a Los Angeles chiropractor who has a special interest in headache patients.

A holistic practitioner, Dr. Pearlman believes that patients should learn to help themselves at home as much as possible and, therefore, taught us both how to stretch neck muscles with towel traction. Here is how it works:

Have the patient lie on her back on the floor. Roll up a bath towel lengthwise. Slip the towel under the patient's neck. Grasp one end of the towel in each hand and, standing behind the patient's head, pull slowly, steadily upward and then back, as in Fig. 2. (Barbara leans back on her heels so she can pull with the full weight of her body.) Lower the head gently to the floor. Do this three times in succession.

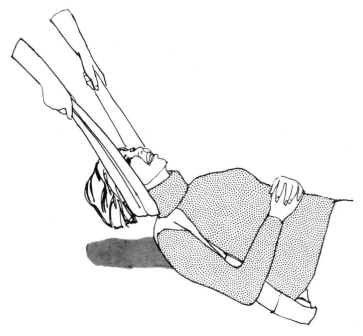

Figure 2

Warning: Don't do towel traction unless you check with your doctor to make sure you don't have some kind of condition (like a broken neck!) that towel traction could worsen. Muscle expert Dr. Rubin says, "Manipulation is not a tool to be played with." And that holds true for traction as well.

Dr. Pearlman also reports success in treating muscle tension headache sufferers by having them sleep on a therapeutic flotation support—a kind of water-filled, two-inch thick mini-mattress placed under the body from about the shoulders to the knees. This alleviates stress and strain on the body and helps avoid muscle contractions that might cause headaches. These flotation supports cost around $35. If you suspect your headaches may be a result of back, shoulder, and neck tension you might want to experiment with one of these. If you can't find a flotation support in your area, you can write to Dr. Pearlman at 5427 Sepulveda Boulevard, Culver City, CA 90230.

## HORMONAL SWORDS
### Female Hormones

As we have already suggested, increased hormonal levels often trigger headaches in women. Some women have to go to the hospital because of headaches during *every* menstrual period. This of course is the extreme. But many women at one age or another have experienced the premenstrual tension headache. Dr. Frederic Speer, an allergist, found that in 14 percent of all cases of women with "migraine," the attacks were regularly associated with menstruation.

Other fascinating facts from the annals of hormonal medicine are that during pregnancy a chronic sufferer may find she has no headaches (not that we're recommending pregnancy as a cure). On the other hand, she may find she has a headache throughout her pregnancy. Menopause is a little more consistent. Headaches of the vascular kind, usually diagnosed by doctors as migraine, decrease or disappear unless you take female hormones, which, judging from all the adverse reports on them, shouldn't be taken anyway.

Then there's the subject of the Pill. Since it increases the level of the hormone estrogen, it can cause headaches and make existing ones more frequent and more painful. However, you need to go for several months without taking the Pill to discover whether it is *the* cause of headaches, and with the increasingly bad press on the Pill you should drop it anyway—and not into your mouth.

While we're on the subject of contraceptives, we heard of one case in which an IUD caused headaches. The doctor noticed that every time the woman had a headache she also ran a high fever. After much investigation he finally discovered she had a pelvic abscess from her IUD. Every once in a while the abscess would burst open and bacteria would enter her blood stream and cause fever and headache. (Let's hear it for a reliable male contraceptive.)

Probably the best testing you can do in regard to your female hormones is to keep careful track of the relationship between your headaches and your monthly period. (See the following diary chapter for a sample recording setup.) If there seems to be a connection, try to work out a solution with your gynecologist.

## Hypoglycemia: Insulin and Adrenalin Levels

The hormonal problem you hear the most about in connection with headaches is hypoglycemia, the medical term for low blood sugar. What you experience in a state of hypoglycemia can include nervousness, depression, irritability, weakness, dizziness, lack of coordination, mental confusion, sweating, and headache.

Diabetics who need to take insulin to properly metabolize carbohydrates experience low blood sugar when they don't eat enough carbohydrate to balance their insulin dosage. Like many diabetics, June is an old pro at letting her blood sugar descend to the hypoglycemic level. When this happens she drinks orange juice or eats some other carbohydrate to bring it up to normal again.

By itself, hypoglycemia can also be a chronic ailment, in which the insulin situation is the reverse of that of diabetes. In this case the pancreas shoots out too much insulin, instead of too little as is the case with diabetes, and keeps the blood sugar level abnormally low. This condition, which is very difficult to diagnose correctly, is controlled by a diet of frequent small meals with emphasis on protein.

Now if you suffer from neither diabetes nor chronic hypoglycemia you still have to become aware of low blood sugar states because they can trigger headaches. In fact, every headache sufferer is advised to avoid low blood sugar. Even if you are not diabetic or hypoglycemic, you can get low blood sugar if you exercise too much or eat too infrequently or do both of these. The remedy is the same as for diabetics: eat or drink some carbohydrate. Some women bring on low blood sugar through poor eating habits—large doses of junk food with high sugar content and then meal skipping to lose weight. Sometimes all you have to do to eliminate hypoglycemic-type headaches is to develop a new eating pattern of regular, frequent, small nutritious meals.

Another variation on the low-blood-sugar blues is the result of living in a stress pattern that gives you low-blood-sugar headaches on weekends only. For example, your regular job may cause a lot of tension because you have an impossible boss or overwhelming demands of some kind. As a reaction to this stress, Monday through Friday your adrenal glands shoot out excessive adrenalin. Adrenalin brings about the body's normal fight-or-flight response (our ancestors' natural reaction to danger) which, in turn, causes the liver to send out its stored sugar. The sugar is energy fuel to help you meet the crisis that stimulated the release of adrenalin. Since usually no real fight or flight is possible and since the extra energy fuel isn't used, you get high blood sugar. To normalize the blood sugar the body responds naturally, with the pancreas releasing insulin into the blood stream. Down goes your blood sugar. This cycle of high-to-low blood sugar repeats itself all during the week.

Then comes the weekend and you relax. Your body is suddenly out from under its usual tension and your adrenal glands slow their pace. But the pancreas hasn't slowed down as quickly as the rest of you. It's still working overtime to bring your adrenalin-induced high blood sugar down. It's still shooting out an overabundance of insulin. Result: The insulin drastically lowers your blood sugar and on Saturday and Sunday you have a low-blood-sugar headache.

If you are trapped in this cycle as a weekend and holiday headachoholic, then you can try to control your headaches by correcting your weekend blood sugar level. According to Dr. Pearlman, the Los Angeles chiropractor, you do this by eating something every half hour for a two-hour period. Begin eating as soon as the headache starts, or if you're really suspicious, start eating before a headache comes on. Dr. Pearlman recommends a piece of fruit, especially an apple, plus a little protein (an ounce of cheese, a thin slice of ham, some peanut butter, etc.).

If eating in this manner every half hour for two hours cures your headache and keeps it away, you may have solved your mystery. An internist or endocrinologist can send you to a lab for a glucose tolerance test to find out exactly what is happening with your blood sugar level.

## VITAMIN AND MINERAL SWORDS
### Vitamins

Vitamins are a double-edged sword: They can give you headaches and they can take away headaches. To launch your investigation into which is the sharper edge in your case, you have to do one of two things. If you are taking large doses of vitamins, stop taking them for four weeks and see whether your headaches diminish. If on the other hand you do not take vitamins or take only minimal potencies of them, start yourself on the high dose of C and B that Dr. Heuser prescribed for June and see if your headache pattern changes. (Some of you may find your headaches get *worse*.)

In the first case—eliminating your regular vitamins—if your headache disappears it may be that the nicotinic acid (niacin) in your B-complex has been triggering headaches, providing your headaches are of the vascular type. One woman who had been prescribed vitamins by two different physicians and was taking a multivitamin on her own had to be hospitalized with excruciating headache pain because of an overdose of nicotinic acid.

As for the second instance—taking megavitamins—some women can cure their headaches in the following manner. You take one high-dosage C (500 milligrams) and one high-dosage B-complex (100 milligrams of almost every component) after each of your three meals. If the vitamins seem to relieve your headaches after you've built up to your headache elimination point, try going two or three days without vitamins and see if your headaches return. This is a good way of confirming whether the vitamins have relieved your headaches. Once you return to the vitamins, the headaches will go away again in only a few days.

No one knows exactly why vitamins are so crucial in some cases. Dr. Heuser theorizes that high C and B in combination serve as a muscle relaxant.

The only problem with taking these megavitamins over a long period of time is that, in some people, they can cause temporary liver damage. If you alert your doctor to what you're doing he can perform a simple blood test to make certain you're not one of the people susceptible to vitamin-induced liver problems.

The 500 milligram C vitamins are easy to find at cut-rate prices in cut-rate pharmacies. And according to Dr. Linus Pauling, that great vitamin C buff who claims C cures the common cold, the C vitamins made in the laboratory by chemists are equally as effective as Mother Nature's. So buy the ones with rose hips if you like, but you'll get a lower price and just as much action out of the nonrosehip variety.

The mega-B 100's are harder to find and exorbitantly priced. June's doctor prescribed the B-complex manufactured by Arco Pharmaceuticals, Inc. (105 Orville Drive, Bohemia, NY 11716). Later she found some other brands in health food stores at a lower price (there's a unique twist for you). We're going to reprint the Arco list of ingredients for you so that you can compare it with whatever brand you find available locally.

### Arco Mega-B

| | |
|---|---:|
| $B_1$ (Thiamine Mononitrate) | 100 mg |
| $B_2$ (Riboflavin) | 60 mg |
| $B_6$ (Pyradoxine hydrocholoride) | 100 mg |
| $B_{12}$ (Cyanocobalamin) | 100 mg |
| Niacinamide | 100 mg |
| Folic Acid | 100 mg |
| Pantothenic Acid | 100 mg |
| Biotin | 100 mcg |
| Para-Aminobenzoic Acid (PABA) | 100 mg |

*Courtesy of Arco Pharmaceuticals, Inc.*

One of the health food brands is Nature's Plus, which contains the same ingredients, except that it has 100 mg of $B_2$ (riboflavin) and only 30 mg of Para-Aminobenzoic acid (PABA). In addition the Nature's Plus pill contains Choline and Inositol.

## Minerals

Along with vitamins, minerals are a double-edged sword. Both deficiencies and excesses can contribute to headaches. The only accurate way to find out your own particular vitamin and mineral deficiencies or excesses is to have an analysis done of your hair. Hair testing is valuable in diagnosis because it tells the story of your health over a long period of time, whereas a blood test only reports on your condition at the instant it was taken. For instance, an M.D. reported to us that he often found large amounts of lead in hair but not in blood.

Unfortunately, women's hair can be so altered by bleaches, dyes, permanents, hair spray, and curlers that it becomes an unreliable indicator. For example, test results on women who had been using aluminum foil to wrap their hair for streaking showed an excess of aluminum. To avoid such problems some doctors use pubic hair for testing.

Because the results of hair testing are so difficult to interpret, it has to be done through a physician and even they sometimes have trouble. If your doctor doesn't have a laboratory in which to do this kind of analysis, you can give him the address of Doctor's Data, a laboratory that does this analysis for doctors by mail (Doctor's Data, Inc., c/o Bio Medical Data, Inc., P.O. Box 397, West Chicago, IL 60185).

Dr. David Bresler of the UCLA Pain Control Unit told us a memorable story involving a mineral excess in one woman with headaches. He had sent a sample of her hair to a laboratory for vitamin and mineral analysis. When the report came back, it indicated such a high concentration of lead that Dr. Bresler thought the lab had made a mistake. But just to check things out he asked the woman if she had anything to do with lead. No, she didn't think so. She thought again and decided, "Oh, yes, I *do* make stained glass windows and do soldering with lead." It turned out she'd been eating without washing her hands after working and was suffering from lead poisoning. She started washing her hands before eating and the headaches disappeared.

Supplements of certain minerals that are purported to help headache sufferers can give some women relief. Among these are lithium, iron, calcium, and iodine. Zinc has also been getting particularly good press lately, and one of the Valley College headache underground members found it quite effective. You might, after getting an OK from your doctor, experiment with these.

## CHEMICAL SWORDS

There's a well-known book we're acquainted with as librarians called *The Chemical Feast*. It's a Nader Study Group report about dangerous chemicals we're exposed to in foods—both knowingly and unknowingly—in present-day U.S.A. From reading this book and others like it and from our own personal experience with drugs and what they do and don't do to you, we've become so concerned about poisoning ourselves that we never buy anything without reading the contents label. And we prepare almost everything we eat from natural (as untampered-with as you can get) products, and June now virtually refuses to take any medicinal drugs.

Paranoid? No, just enlightened. It's almost impossible to avoid a certain number of hazardous swipes from the chemical swords of our additive-addicted culture. The best we can do is give you a general beware and then touch on a few specific examples that are directly related to headaches.

### MSG (Monosodium Glutamate)

MSG, which is used extensively in Chinese cookery, is probably *the* most famous headache-inducing chemical. It dilates blood vessels and people who are susceptible to MSG get a headache twenty to thirty minutes after eating three grams of it on an empty stomach—the amount in a seven-ounce bowl of wonton soup.

Doctors call the MSG headache "the Chinese restaurant syndrome." According to Dr. James W. Lance, an Australian neurologist, you can sidestep it to a certain extent, if you are susceptible, by skipping the soup in a Chinese restaurant and eating food first. In certain Chinese restaurants where the food is cooked to order, you can request that they leave the MSG out. But if we were you and had this tendency, we'd cook our own Chinese food at home without any MSG.

The real problem is that it's not just Chinese restaurants that like the flavor-enhancing capabilities of MSG. American food processors in general are in love with it. If you don't believe us, read the labels on frozen dinners, canned and bottled anythings, and watch ham and bacon, too, because some brands are cured with MSG and/or soy sauce. (Soy sauce contains MSG as does Accent.)

**Nitrates and Nitrites**

Sodium nitrate is the culprit in the "hot dog headache." Nitrates and nitrites are used to preserve or cure meats—hot dogs, bacon, ham, salami, corned beef, and other deli items—poultry, and fish and in some cases to give these foods their red coloring.

If food processors cannot prove these chemicals are safe (that is, not carcinogenic or cancer producing) they will be prohibited by the FDA. But these government prohibitions are usually slow in coming. Also, the FDA usually has to give the manufacturers time to use up the supply of the harmful chemical they have on hand. That's what is known as the American way to do business.

Dr. Frederick J. Hass, author of *What You Can Do About Headaches*, says a man told him that if you boil hot dogs, the nitrate is removed, and you can't get a "hot dog headache" from them. (Ten to one that man worked for a meat packing firm.)

## Caffeine

Caffeine is a blood vessel constrictor and, especially in combination with aspirin or ergotamine preparations, can help alleviate headache pain. But caffeine also does the opposite with some people—it precipitates headaches. It is addictive and, if you're a heavy user (up to fifteen cups of coffee a day) and try to kick the habit, you can get a withdrawal headache, called a "rebound headache" by doctors.

Since caffeine constricts the blood vessels in the head (as well as everywhere else), heavy coffee drinkers go around with semiconstricted blood vessels all the time. Then when they let up a bit—say, sleep late on Saturday or Sunday mornings and miss their early coffee—the blood vessels, without their usual coffee fix, dilate. This swelling of the vessels inside the head causes a headache. If you are a heavy caffeine imbiber, you can try to give it up for two or three weeks and see if your headache goes away and stays away.

Coffee is not the sole supplier of caffeine. Cola drinks, tea, chocolate, and some aspirin combinations like Midol and other drugs contain varying amounts of caffeine. To do an adequate caffeine test, you have to eliminate it *entirely*. So consult the following chart before starting the experiment and, again, read labels on everything.

### Caffeine Content of Beverages

| Beverage | Milligrams Caffeine per Ounce |
|---|---|
| Decaffeinated coffee | 0.6 to 1.6 |
| Chocolate drinks | 1.0 to 2.5 |

| | |
|---|---|
| Cola | 2.4 to 5.3 |
| Iced tea mixes | 2.4 to 6.9 |
| Black tea<br>    brewed 1 minute | 4.2 to 7.7 |
| Tea (other than black)<br>    brewed 3-5 minutes | 4.2 to 8.8 |
| Black tea<br>    brewed 3-5 minutes | 7.0 to 13.2 |
| Instant coffee | 11.6 to 14.0 |
| Percolator coffee | 18.0 to 25.0 |
| Dripolator coffee | 27.0 to 29.4 |

## Alcohol

Alcohol expands the blood vessels and is particularly a hazard for women who get vascular headaches. Many people have an intolerance to alcohol or to some of the substances in it. Dr. Frederic Speer, the allergist, says, "This is especially true of women." Different liquors have different chemicals (amines) to give them their distinctive flavors and to give you your distinctive headache. Vodka is the purest type of alcoholic beverage and from this point of view the safest.

You can have allergies to the corn in whiskeys, the hops in beers, or the grapes in wine. If you're suspicious of any form of alcohol and its role in your headaches, why not go on the wagon for a few weeks and see what happens or doesn't happen? Remember the case we cited earlier about the beer drinker with "laughing headaches."

In bringing up alcohol as a possible culprit, we're not considering it in the usual context of the hangover headache. A hangover is what you might call a "normal headache." Anyone can get one by overimbibing. You of course can get them, too, but hangover headaches are the simplest kind to prevent and the solution is equally simple: moderation in all things alcoholic.

## Tyramine

Tyramine is a food chemical (an amine) that dilates blood vessels and, as we have been discovering, anything that alters blood vessels can alter the way you feel in the head. Found mainly in aged cheeses and red wines, tyramine has been the subject of several studies (none definitive) because it may be a headache trigger.

Since it was impossible to find a good list of tyramine-high foods in any one place, we went to several lists in library books and scientific journals. Here is the most complete chart we can give you.

### Tyramine-High Foods

Dairy Products: Aged cheeses—cheddar, Gruyère, Stilton, Emmentaler, Brie, Camembert, Gouda, mozzarella, Parmesan, provolone, romano, Roquefort, Swiss, edam; yogurt, sour cream

Meats and Fish: Pickled herring, salted dried fish, sausages, beef, and chicken liver

Vegetables: Italian broad beans with pods (fava beans), sauerkraut

Other: Vanilla, chocolate, yeast and yeast extracts, soy sauce

Alcoholic Beverages: Beer, ale, red wines (chianti is the worst), Riesling, sauterne, champagne, sherry

To perform a valid tyramine test, eliminate all these foods at the same time for two to four weeks and see if your headaches go away.

## Drugs

According to one headache therapist we talked to, if you exclude antibiotics, 90 percent of the drugs listed in the

*PDR (Physician's Desk Reference)* have headaches as one of their side effects. It could then be that some drug you take for a condition as far removed from your head as, say, hemorrhoids, is one of the triggering factors for your headaches. It's a sound practice to look up whatever you're taking in the *PDR* and see if you get any good headache leads.

One word of caution: A UCLA pharmacist said that if a drug is ever known to produce headaches in even the most minute sampling of subjects, headache has to be listed as a side effect in the *PDR*. Often it is a very rare side effect. Consequently, if you do find headache listed for a drug you're taking, don't immediately jump to the happy conclusion that you've found the cause and hence the cure for your headache.

Another problem with drugs is that the medication you're taking to alleviate your headache, if abused, can contribute to the headache. Painkilling drugs blunt the body's system of coping with pain and the more you incapacitate your own natural pain-inhibitory mechanism the more pain you feel. Doctors refer to people caught up in this trap as "analgesic junkies." Often they have to hospitalize such patients to get them off their drug. Ironically, sometimes just withdrawing all their analgesics relieves their pain.

One more case in which the cure for the malady can become its cause is the combination of aspirin and vitamin C. Vitamin C prolongs and intensifies the action of aspirin. This can be a desirable thing, but in certain people it can also produce the side effects of dizziness and (what else?) headaches.

## Nicotine

Can cigarettes, those coffin nails of emphysema and cancer fame, also cause hammering in your head? Yes. In fact, you don't even have to be a smoker yourself. You just have to sit in the proverbial smoke-filled room or breathe someone's sidestream smoke to become an innocent victim.

If you are a smoker, we hope you know that nicotine is another blood vessel shrinker. Not only can it be a headache trigger, but as with caffeine, you can get a rebound headache if you forego your habitual quota. Frankly, we are antismoking bigots and can't muster up much sympathy for anyone who smokes, especially not for a headachoholic who smokes. We will grant this, however: We've read that it is more difficult to kick an addiction to nicotine than an addiction to heroin. We hope, however, you won't use that as an excuse.

## ENVIRONMENTAL SWORDS

In this category we wish we could give you the definitive environmental impact statement to apply to your headache problem. That, unfortunately, is impossible. Not even the most detailed government-financed study could begin to cover all the negative elements that now assault us from without. Therefore, we are of necessity limiting ourselves to those environmental swords that have a direct and proven history of wounding the head: altitude, wind and weather, and air pollution.

### Altitude

Some people, and this time it's Barbara instead of June who's one of them, can expect a splitting headache whenever they suddenly go to altitudes over 6,000 feet. The altitude headache, some believe, comes from breathing air containing less oxygen than your body is accustomed to, causing concomitant swelling of the arteries in the scalp. Another theory is that these headaches result from hyperventilation, that is, you breathe too rapidly in order to extract the diminished oxygen from the air. This causes you to lose too much carbon dioxide and the lack of carbon dioxide brings on the headache.

Whichever the problem is, oxygen or carbon dioxide, these headaches can often be prevented by approaching the higher altitude in slow stages and avoiding exertion the first few days up there. But that's usually impossible in ski and mountain resort vacations, especially weekend ones. Barbara's technique is to avoid alcohol, take aspirin, and suffer. You may prefer complete abstinence from high altitudes, especially if your tendency is toward vascular headaches.

It is also fairly well established that another altitude factor, a sudden change in air pressure by going either higher or lower, can trigger headaches. But then we have another of those paradoxes we find so often in headache detection circles: these same changes in pressure can sometimes break up a headache. For example, June's week-long headache lifted the moment the airplane to Europe did. On the other end of the air pressure (or water) scale, one headache patient can almost invariably abort an incipient sinus headache by diving into her pool and sitting on the bottom.

## Wind and Weather

Some old folks say they can predict a rain storm by a flare-up of their lumbago or pain in their joints. This is not all in their minds but in their bodies, too. Changes in humidity and in barometric pressure *do* affect your body, and especially those of you with vascular headaches. June, you may recall, found she had fewer headaches in cool, damp weather. Other women react in the dead opposite manner to damp weather. They *get* headaches. Along with changes in humidity, drops in barometric pressure, especially when there's another contributing factor (food, ovulation, stress, etc.), can trigger a headache.

The weather phenomenon most notorious in headache circles is what are known as "hot winds of ill repute." Here in Southern California our wind of ill repute is the Santa

Ana (sometimes also called Santana), which are winds originating in the desert. The weather conditions associated with these hot winds are a decrease in humidity to below 25 to 30 percent, an increase in temperature, and a preliminary period of high levels of positive ions (electrical charges) in the air.

Ions are either positive or negative, but it is the lack of negative ones that is most detrimental to health. The particular effect of breathing negative-ion-poor air is a drop in the body's oxygen level and an increase in the serotonin level. (Serotonin is a chemical that constricts the blood vessels.) The result may be sleepiness, fatigue, inability to concentrate, depression, respiratory ailments, and headaches.

This brings us to a subject which may be a new one to you, the problem of negative-ion-poor air in big cities and urban environments. It is in Europe that air ionization and its effect on human health have been studied the most.

The only information we found about treating headaches by exposure to negative ions came to us from Dr. Albert Paul Krueger, M.D., a research biometeorologist, at the University of California, Berkeley. Though Dr. Krueger himself has done research only on plants and small animals, his reports from the field include one from Dr. Peter Fox of Dorchester, Dorset, England, who personally suffered from migraines and eventually prevented them by exposure to negative ions in the air. In his medical practice Dr. Fox has conducted investigations over a number of years with migraine patients and has found that in selected cases (certain types) of migraine he gets some 90 percent of "cures."

Dr. Krueger sent us his list of American manufacturers of negative air ion generators, which you can buy for use in your home, though he cautioned that this kind of equipment cannot be sold in interstate commerce within the U.S.A. if any health claims are made for it. The cost of these machines probably varies considerably, but to give you a ball-park figure, we heard one advertised on a San Francisco radio station for slightly under $100.

**Negative Ion Generator Manufacturers**
Amcor Group, P.O. Box 978, Edison, NJ
DEV Industries Inc., 5721 Arapahoe, Boulder, CO 80302
Omega Systems, P.O. Box 601, San Leandro, CA 94577
Pro Team Associates, 4425 Carson, Oakland, CA 94619

Also, if you're adept at electronics or know someone who is, there are directions for building a generator in the June, 1971 issue of *Radio Electronics*.

If you live in an area where the negative ion level is low or where there are "hot winds of ill repute," you might keep your eyes open for further research reports about the effects of these phenomena on health in general and headaches in particular. Or, you might consider acquiring a generator. Since negative ions have been called "the vitamins of the air," they could make a difference in how you feel and in how many headaches you get.

## Air Pollution

It is almost universally agreed that air pollution can trigger vascular headaches and can increase the frequency and severity of any kind of headache. (We still believe it wasn't just coincidental that June's headaches were more frequent and severe in high smog periods.) The problem is believed to be caused by the build-up of carbon monoxide along with a decrease in the body's ability to absorb oxygen because of the other contaminants in the air. (And speaking of other contaminants, one of these, ozone, is a notorious headache causer. Passengers and crews of airlines flying through areas with high ozone levels complain that they develop "migraine" headaches.)

The most depressing aspect of air pollution is that there is very little you can do about it, except move out of the smog area, as June did over and over again. This is not only expensive and impractical, but the air pollution is very likely to follow wherever you go. Smog is almost becoming the earth's natural air these days.

You should certainly listen to and read the air pollution reports. When the levels are high and, as the Los Angeles report puts it, "unhealthful for sensitive people," stay indoors as much as possible.

Some vitamin advocates maintain that vitamin E helps you withstand the smog better by increasing your ability to extract oxygen from air garbage. It wouldn't hurt, therefore, to increase your intake of vitamin E during periods of high smog.

Finally, you might do as we do for more reasons than smog avoidance. Spend all your vacations away from cities so that at least once in a while you can breathe the few quarts of clean air that are left on the planet.

## STRESS SWORDS

Without the swords of stress it's doubtful that you could feel the thrust of any of the others. Stress slashes away all your physical and psychological armor against headaches and leaves you wide open to attack from all sides. You may feel we're overplaying our hand—or our sword—here, but there's more than enough scientific data to back up the most extravagant-sounding statements about the detrimental effects of stress. Social and medical scientists estimate that between 60 and 85 percent of our diseases are now stress induced. The four major ailments of the seventies—cardiovascular disease, cancer, arthritis, and respiratory disease—have all burgeoned because of the immense stressfulness of modern life.

We might ask at this point, why did you get headaches instead of one of these other problems? The great Canadian stress authority, Dr. Hans Selye, says it's because "in the body, as in a chain, the weakest link breaks down under stress, although all parts are equally exposed." Your head is apparently your weakest link. To keep this vulnerable area from breaking down, you have to learn how to assess your stresses and then do something about them.

Many of us are not clear about what stress really is. If we have a close call on the freeway, we recognize the pounding heart, the rapid breathing, the cold hands and realize that a physiological reaction has taken place. Or consider an entirely different kind of threat, one that seems psychological. Picture yourself waiting to be interviewed for a job you really need and want. Are there physical sensations similar to those of the freeway incident? Yes, of course.

Our responses to these two patently visible threats are clear to us, expected and rational. But many of the stresses we're talking about here are invisible to us and by that very token more insidious. They produce exactly the same chemicals, hormones, and muscle spasms that cause the physical reactions we experience during recognizable challenges to our safety and well-being. But we take no notice.

In this section we're going to give you some good techniques for analyzing and recognizing pressures in your life. And since stress is the one sword you have the most personal control over, in Chapter 7 we'll go into detail about ways of controlling and removing it.

## Life Changes

Any life change can bring on stress. A normal event that causes you to have to change or adapt to new situations or any alteration in your life that requires you to adjust is a stressor. The important stressors are pregnancy, marriage, divorce, death, graduation, retirement, a vacation, a new job, a new apartment (not necessarily in order of importance).

Selye uses the terms *distress* and *eustress* to differentiate between stress that gives rise to bad feelings (a divorce) and stress that gives rise to good feelings (a vacation). It doesn't matter whether the change is for the better or worse. If you make too many changes in your life too quickly and too frequently without enough time for recovery, you undergo a damaging stress reaction. In your case this can mean the water behind your dam gets so high that it spills over into headaches.

The discovery that pleasurable as well as unpleasurable activities of life underlie much illness was made by two researchers at the University of Washington in Seattle. Thomas H. Holmes and Richard H. Rahe devised a chart and point scale of stressful life happenings. To use the chart, check off events that have happened to you within the last year and then total the score by adding the assigned values. If your score is 150, you have a fifty-fifty chance of developing an illness or maybe accentuating one you already have. A score of over 300 indicates a 90 percent chance for illness. Viewed holistically, it's not the individual events but the cluster that causes your resistance to disease to be lowered, just as it's the cluster of contributing factors that builds up to headaches.

You might find a direct connection between your headaches and stress by calculating what your chances of developing an illness were according to this chart the year before you became a chronic headache sufferer.

### Social Readjustment Rating Scale

| Event | Value |
|---|---|
| Death of spouse | 100 |
| Divorce | 73 |
| Marital separation | 65 |
| Jail term | 63 |
| Death of close family member | 63 |
| Personal injury or illness | 53 |
| Marriage | 50 |
| Fired from work | 47 |
| Marital reconciliation | 45 |

Retirement .............................  45
Change in family member's health ........  44
Pregnancy .............................  40
Sex difficulties .........................  39
Addition to family ......................  39
Business readjustment ...................  39
Change in financial status ...............  38
Death of close friend ...................  37
Change to different line of work ..........  36
Change in number of marital arguments ...  35
Mortgage or loan over $10,000 ...........  31
Foreclosure of mortgage or loan ..........  30
Change in work responsibilities ...........  29
Son or daughter leaving home ............  29
Trouble with in-laws ....................  29
Outstanding personal achievement ........  28
Spouse begins or stops work .............  26
Starting or finishing school ..............  26
Change in living conditions ..............  25
Revision of personal habits ...............  24
Trouble with boss ......................  23
Change in work hours, conditions ........  20
Change in residence ....................  20
Change in schools ......................  20
Change in recreational habits .............  19
Change in church activities ...............  19
Change in social activities ................  18
Mortgage or loan under $10,000 ..........  17
Change in sleeping habits ................  16
Change in number of family gatherings ....  15
Change in eating habits ..................  15
Vacation ..............................  13
Christmas season .......................  12
Minor violation of the law ...............  11

*Courtesy of Thomas H. Holmes, M.D., Professor of Psychiatry and Behavioral Sciences, University of Washington, Seattle, Washington.*

## Body Signals

Besides monitoring your life changes for stress, you can also watch your body patterns. Our bodies give off signals when they're tense. Learn these signals and you'll know when you'd better start doing something about the tightness, tension, and anxiety you're exhibiting.

> **Breathing.** The best indicator of what's going on inside you. Often the very first sign. Short and shallow means tension; holding your breath means extreme tension.
>
> **Muscle stiffness and aching.** Reflect tightness and gripping over long periods of time. Head, neck, shoulder, and upper back muscles are most involved. When you grip hard you often tighten the fist, hunch the shoulders, or clench the jaw.
>
> **Warmth.** Overworked nerves create heat; you may even perspire under too much pressure, literally "break into a sweat."
>
> **Fatigue.** Anxiety and frustration cause exhaustion, even though you do nothing strenuous physically. Emotions, especially bottled-up emotions, are the problem, not overwork.

## THE TMJ SWORD

Now we come to the supersword, a veritable Excalibur. The temporomandibular joint syndrome (TMJ) sword is the equivalent of all the basic seven swords rolled into one because if you are pierced by this sword and it alone is pulled out, your headaches go away. Sometimes they disappear within twenty-four hours; sometimes it takes a few weeks or months, as in June's case, but they *do* go. It seems like magic, a miracle.

The problem with the TMJ sword, however, is like that of the original Excalibur: You have to find some King Arthur among physicians or dentists who has the perspicacity to get a handle on it and pull it out for you.

The TMJ syndrome is a medical problem that must be treated by a dentist who is a specialist. A further complication, according to Dr. Victor Mintz, former director of the TMJ clinic at the UCLA School of Dentistry, is that it is a "grossly overlooked condition."

He compares looking for a TMJ dysfunction in a patient to hunting for elephants. If you don't have any idea what an elephant looks like, you can see a whole herd of them and yet come back from your safari and report "I didn't see an elephant the whole time." Dentists who don't know what the TMJ dysfunction is (and this is the vast majority of dentists) never see it in their patients.

A dentist who *does* know "sees the elephant" in about 20 percent of the mouths he examines. According to Dr. Douglas Morgan, another Southern California dentist who specializes in TMJ, that's the percentage of the population that suffers from TMJ. Not all of these sufferers have chronic headaches, but Dr. Morgan believes that as many as 50 percent of chronic headache sufferers possibly do have the TMJ problem.

A large majority of these TMJ headache victims are women. In the dental literature we've read that TMJ patients are usually "neurotic women"—young and unmarried, married to weak husbands whom they dominate, or menopausal. Dr. Morgan says that, indeed, about 90 percent of his TMJ patients are women. Dr. Mintz puts his figure at 80 percent although he adds, "Eighty percent of *all* my patients are women. Women take better care of their teeth and more of them come into the office."

Dr. Mintz discounts the idea that most TMJ patients are neurotic. He says that one dentist reported this years ago and though there is no justification for it, each generation of dental students has been taught the same mistake. Then, too, there is always the problem that long-term chronic pain can make a person neurotic. It's only normal to get a little neurotic after years of hurting and having everyone tell you that it's all in your mind.

All experts agree, however, that emotion and stress enter into the TMJ picture. A person can have the condition for years and not even know it until some tension-producing life situation brings out the headache pain.

## The Great Imposter

TMJ is not only frequently overlooked, it is just as frequently misdiagnosed. This is because, as Dr. Morgan wrote in the *Journal of the American Medical Association*, it is "the great imposter presenting one of the most baffling diagnostic problems encountered by the medical and dental profession...these [TMJ] patients go from doctor to doctor with a multitude of seemingly unrelated symptoms...there may be pain that resembles a migraine, sinus problems, atypical facial pain mimicking a tic douloureux or a temporal arteritis, or neck and shoulder pain..."

TMJ is especially clever at imitating migraine. A TMJ victim can have almost every one of the classic migraine symptoms of nausea, unilateral pain, and visual changes.

Once the TMJ headache sufferer has overcome the hurdle of correct diagnosis, as June did after five years, what are the techniques and possibilities for a cure? Most specialists begin with splint (plane) therapy, as Dr. Greene did for June. The splint gives 75 percent of the people relief by correcting the position of the muscles around the joint. (Actually TMJ is a misnomer. The problem, according to Dr. Mintz, is not in the joint but in the muscles around it, and both he and Dr. Greene prefer to call it the TM syndrome.)

After three to twelve weeks and when the patient has relief signs, the bite is permanently corrected to the new position by grinding down the teeth or putting in crowns. The splint is only a crutch and should be followed up with long-range correction.

It is possible, however, if you have neither the time nor the money for further dental work (remember June's

$4,200 bill), to use holistic, self-regulatory techniques to avoid pain. One of Dr. Mintz's patients who couldn't afford a permanent cure would put in the splint when she felt herself building toward a headache and made a conscious effort not to clench her teeth. She would also escape for a while from her demanding family until she could feel the stress-induced tension slip away and her muscles relax.

In some cases patients have destruction in the joint itself—osteoarthritis, for example. An oral surgeon can replace the damaged joint with a metal reconstruction, but as Dr. Mintz admonishes, "The surgical approach to joints has to be the last approach."

## Checking Out the Joint

In the meantime, what do you do to find out if TMJ might be the cause or a contributing factor to your headaches? First, check yourself on this list of symptoms and tests that we have compiled from Dr. Morgan's TMJ questionnaire for patients, from the diagnostic techniques in Dr. Mintz's lecture to doctors at a headache seminar, and from those tests Dr. Greene and Dr. Heuser performed on June or had her perform on herself. Some of the following symptoms may appear to be so unrelated to the jaw that they don't make sense to you unless you are aware that the TMJ syndrome sets up disturbances in muscles and nerves that affect the whole body. The whys behind certain of the TMJ symptoms included here are still not totally understood by physicians and dentists. Their inclusion is based on clinical evidence (experience with patients).

1. Do you have pain in any of the following areas: In the temporomandibular joint itself, in the lower jaw, in the upper jaw, in the neck, in the shoulders, in the forehead, in the facial muscles, behind the eyes, in the temple, in the tongue?
2. Do you have a grating, clicking, cracking, or popping sound in the joint when you chew?

3. Do you ever have a ringing, roaring, or hissing sound in your ears?
4. Do you sometimes have sensations of pressure blockage in your ears?
5. Do you ever feel dizzy or faint?
6. Do you sometimes have an upset stomach or nausea for no apparent reason?
7. Do you perspire excessively?
8. Do you usually feel sluggish and irritable when you wake up in the morning?
9. Do you always feel fatigued in the late afternoon?
10. Do you sometimes have a tingling in your fingers?
11. Do you have a speech defect, especially a lisp?
12. Do you put your tongue between your teeth when you swallow?
13. Is one leg shorter than the other? (See test in Postural Swords section.)
14. Have you ever worn a cervical collar?
15. Do you have difficulty moving your jaw from left to right or forward and backward?
16. Do you usually finish eating either way before or way after everybody else? (People with TMJ often either give up trying to chew effectively and just swallow their food whole, or they have such difficulty chewing that it takes them a long time to finish.)
17. Do you have any missing teeth?
18. Have you ever worn braces on your teeth?
19. Have you had extensive dental reconstruction? (Note: If you did, try to remember if your headaches began shortly afterward.)
20. Do you sometimes find yourself clenching your teeth?
21. Has anyone ever told you that you grind your teeth in your sleep?
22. Do you usually have to get up several times in the night to urinate? (One of Dr. Greene's patients had

to get up ten to twelve times a night before her TMJ syndrome was corrected.)

23. Do you have excessive ear wax?
24. Do you frequently wake up with a headache?
25. Have you ever had a whiplash injury? (According to Dr. Mintz, 99 percent of these result in the TMJ syndrome.)
26. Have you ever had a blow to the chin, face, or head in an accident (contact sports, falling off a bicycle or horse, automobile accident, etc.)?
27. Are your headaches usually not helped by drugs? (Aspirin is the only one that seems to help at all. This is because it has a cortisone-like effect in reducing muscle pain.)

Count how many yes answers you had to the above questions. How many does it take to indicate TMJ syndrome? Well, for what it's worth, June would have had seventeen yes's. But as Dr. Greene said, she was an extreme case. Actually, these questions are like the ones on those "Are you an alcoholic?" quizzes that magazines are always running. Any yes answer at all is a danger signal. Therefore, if you have any yes answers at all, it would be worth your while to try the following tests.

1. Sometimes when you *don't* have a headache, chew a wad of bubblegum for a couple of hours or eat a large box of popcorn to see if you can bring on a headache.
2. Sometime when you *do* have a headache, see if you can cure it by holding half a popsicle stick or tongue depressor between your upper and lower teeth. (You'll have to break it in two in order to fit it into your mouth.) The rationale behind this is that by realigning your jaw you can sometimes ease the problem and make your pain disappear.
3. Press your fingertips hard against the muscles just

in front of your ears and above your jaw joint. Then open and close your mouth. If there is soreness in the muscles, this could indicate that TMJ is at least partially responsible for your headaches. (Although June had soreness when Dr. Greene did this test, she was not able to bring on a headache with the bubblegum or cure one with the popsicle stick.)

4. Stick your index fingers into your ears and pull forward while you open and close your mouth and see if you feel pain or soreness.

5. Look at yourself in a mirror while you open your mouth. Does your jaw go off to either the left or right instead of dropping straight down? (This was one of the diagnostic tests that helped reveal June's TMJ syndrome to Dr. Greene. Her jaw went off to the left side in an exaggerated way.)

6. Open your mouth as wide as you can and see if you can insert the first three knuckles of your hand. If you can't, this could be a TMJ syndrome indication.

7. The most exciting way to check your TMJ possibilities—among other possibilities—is to have a night of passionate kissing and see if you wake up with an immobilized jaw or a headache. This TMJ phenomenon was reported by a University of Toronto dentist at a California Dental Association meeting. Because of the kissing involved, TMJ could be responsible for the so-called "intercourse headache," though some headaches that take place during or after intercourse can be vascular in origin, a result of alterations in the blood flow.

**Final Examination**

If any of these TMJ tests indicates to you that TMJ might be a part of your headache problem, then an official examination is in order. You might first have a frank talk with your dentist, asking him if he's familiar with the TMJ syndrome, or Costen's syndrome, as it was originally called. Should he claim a knowledge of TMJ and assure you that it's no part of your problem, it might behoove you to heed the words of Dr. Mintz: "Even if a well-known dentist tells you that you don't have TMJ, you may want to check further because the dentist may not be aware of the many advances in TMJ diagnosis that have been made in recent years." In other words, your dentist may not be able to "see the elephant."

Since TMJ is essentially a medical problem, perhaps your physician may be familiar with it and know of a dentist to whom he could refer you. Strangely enough, chiropractors are frequently able to diagnose TMJ because they recognize it through the muscle involvement. They also treat it with some success, but the relief is usually temporary because, if the dental problem isn't corrected, the muscle problems are likely to recur.

A partial listing of TMJ specialists and clinics appears in Appendix C. If local sources fail you, you can go national by writing to the following organizations to ask for the names of TMJ specialists in your vicinity:

**American Board of Prosthedontics**
Milton H. Brown, D.D.S.
School of Dentistry
State University of New York at Buffalo
Buffalo, NY 14260

**American Academy of**
**Craniomandibular Orthopedics**
Suite 201
3366 Park Avenue
Wantaugh, NY 11793

**American Equilibration Society**
Malcolm E. Boone, D.D.S., Secretary
4706 Melbourne Road
Indianapolis, IN 46708

# 4

## DIARY
## OF A MAD
## HEADACHE SUFFERER

IF you're going to be able to bring order out of the chaos of clues you unearth with all your tests and experiments, you'll need to keep a personal headache diary. At its best your diary may reveal a significant pattern in the overall picture of your headaches and thereby present you with a simple cure that will allow you to make an immediate quantum leap out of the land of headache pain.

At the very least your diary will be a valuable holistic tool to present to your doctor. The minute mind and body, life and health details that may seem insignificant to you may be exactly the information he needs to bring your headache case to a solution. And it can also provide you with the emotional benefits of being able to confide in an understanding, uncritical therapist with whom you can always get an appointment and who never tells you your time is up.

June started keeping a headache diary before her first appointment with Dr. Heuser, who likes his patients to keep a running account of their headaches and headache-related happenings. Until she began her diary keeping, June really knew very little about her headaches. She didn't even know how often she had them. It *seemed* she had them all the time and yet she realized she didn't. Merely discovering the frequency by recording her headaches in the diary was a breakthrough.

It's also true that it's hard to think straight when you're hurting. As June said in one of her later journal entries, "Pain induces a kind of intellectual blindness." She found her diary restored her vision and allowed her to see the facts of her situation more clearly.

## STARTING LINES

To start with the basics, we recommend that you buy an inexpensive notebook to be used exclusively for headache journalizing. You can flow better if you don't lock yourself into one of those calendar-style diary or appointment books. These usually allow too few lines per day and always the same number. This causes you to write too small or to omit important information.

It would be best if you got a notebook of a size that you can fit into your purse so you can keep it with you at all times and make notes on meals you have away from home and record miscellaneous events when they take place.

And we recommend using a pen. It's smoother to write with and easier to read.

Now, for when to write. Spreading the writing out over the entire day and jotting down your notes immediately after the fact is the way the best detectives do it. The important feature of this method is that you don't forget vital information. For instance, if you describe how you slept immediately upon awakening, then you're pretty sure to be complete and accurate. With diet and drugs you also have to try to get your facts down immediately or you may not get them down at all.

This brings us to the human factor: excuses. "I had no time," "I was too tired," "I just didn't feel like it," and the unassailable, "I had a headache." These are the excuses we all fall back on when inertia is in control, as it typically is when a person has chronic pain. You've got to fight it, especially in the beginning when resistance is highest. After you've been at it a while, the diary becomes like a friend with whom you're accustomed to having a daily conversation.

Don't worry about being too tired or in too much pain to write. Although it may be difficult to write when you're hurting, it's the only way you can accurately describe what the pain is like. And according to *Los Angeles Times* book critic Robert Kirsch, it's preferable to write in a diary when you're tired because then your defenses are down, poses are out of the way, and the real you comes out.

## OUTLINES

If your diary is going to be the kind of holistic tool that will work for you, it has to be totally subjective in form and content. Therefore, we don't want to lock you into a structure with which you don't feel comfortable. The following is just to give you an idea of what to include and to show you a way of organizing the information.

First we'll give you a general outline of a diary entry and then we'll break down each part into its specifics.

### Outline

1. Date, Day of Week, Place
2. Weather
3. Sleep and Dream Patterns
4. Headache Analysis
5. Special Tests and Test Results
6. The Physiological You: Health and Medications
7. The Psychological You: Stresses and Emotions
8. Diet

9. Activities and Exercise
10. Free-form Ranting
11. Dialogue for Self-Discovery

**1. Date, Day of Week, Place.** You need the day of the week as well as the date in order to see if there is a pattern to your headaches. For example, do they pop up regularly on Mondays or weekends? The place could be significant if you discovered that you, like June, never had a headache when you were away from home or, conversely, always had a headache when you were out of your familiar environment.

**2. Weather.** An easy way to enter the weather facts in your diary is to clip the forecast out of the newspaper, unless it's the usual meteorological misprediction. Be sure to include such weather specifics as humidity, whether or not there are winds (and from what direction they're coming), barometric pressure (some TV weathercasters give this), temperature range, and air pollution. Any of these can be headache inducers.

**3. Sleep and Dream Patterns of the Previous Night.** Cover the night's sleep or nonsleep: the hour at which you went to bed, how many hours you spent awake and when these occurred, number of trips to the bathroom, time you got up in the morning, and whether you felt rested or depleted, amiable or grouchy. Did you dream and, if so, what was the dream? Always try to remember your dreams. If necessary keep a pad and pen beside your bed so you can get them down before you forget them. Your dreams could be telling you something significant about your life—and your headaches.

**4. Headache Analysis.** Paste a small calendar in the front of your diary and circle on it the dates on which you have headaches. This is another way of seeing if there are patterns to your headache. It will look something like this calendar taken from June's diary:

October 17 – November 17

|      | S    | M    | T    | W    | T    | F    | S    |
|------|------|------|------|------|------|------|------|
| Oct. | 17   | 18   | 19   | 20   | 21   | 22   | 23   |
|      | 24   | 25   | 26   | (27) | (28) | (29) | 30   |
| Nov. | (31) | (1)  | (2)  | 3    | 4    | 5    | 6    |
|      | 7    | 8    | 9    | 10   | 11   | 12   | (13) |
|      | 14   | (15) | (16) | 17   |      |      |      |

Then, in your daily entry indicate again if you have a headache. If you do, elaborate, telling at what time it began or ended or what day of its duration it is. Rate its intensity on a scale of one to ten. Tell where the headache is localized, how it feels, and if it's the usual or some new variation of pain or ache. As we said before, try to write while you're actually in pain. It may not be easy to do, but it will be very valuable to you if you can. Nature is very kind about allowing you to forget how pain feels once it's over and you will never be able to describe it as well as you can while it's going on.

If this day is the first day of a headache, describe your activities and physical sensations during the period preceding its development. If you learn to recognize the harbingers of your headaches, you may be able to find ways to head them off.

**5. Special Tests and Test Results.** You will probably be conducting various of the special tests mentioned in Chapter 3 or other tests your doctor has suggested. In this section give the progress reports and results and, if you can, try to relate them to your headache or lack thereof. Here you make notes on clues from food checks, drug checks, special diets (low tyramine, hypoglycemic), vitamins and minerals, and abstinence from alcohol, nicotine, etc. Be sure to mention any cheating you do on tests you're carrying out. June wrote in a Thanksgiving Day entry: "Broke low-tyramine diet with one ounce vodka before dinner and one three-ounce glass rosé wine with dinner, plus two cups of coffee—one in early morning and one in midafternoon."

This is also where you could get into the musculo-skeletal checks and balances: You may mention giving up driving your sports car, changing your typing position at the office, sleeping on your side rather than your stomach, or any of the other muscle tension habits we recommended altering in Chapter 3.

Record, too, the answers from any TMJ checks you're making.

**6. The Physiological You: Health and Medications.** If you have any chronic maladies besides headaches—high blood pressure, diabetes, asthma—report on the state of these. Also, give details on special illnesses and infections like colds, stomach upsets, cuts, burns, and the like—any kind of physical trauma that might conceivably trigger a headache that is ready to go over the dam.

Above all, mention your menstrual cycle and keep close track of it. (Mark it on your calendar in the front of the diary along with your headaches.) Here give details of length, profusion of flow, discomforts, mood changes, any differences from the usual.

Next launch into an exact accounting of the day's drug doses and medications. What did you take and how much? Include everything prescription or nonprescription: birth control pills, estrogen, aspirin or any other painkillers, tranquilizers, vitamins, minerals, alcohol, marijuana, tobacco, and whatever else you're altering your chemistry with.

Mention how you felt *physically*—healthy, energetic, exhausted, achy, nauseated, etc.

**7. The Psychological You: Stresses and Emotions.** Since stress—both distress and eustress—can trigger headaches, it has to occupy a prominent place in the diary. What you need to record in this section are all the highs and lows of your daily life that can act as stressors.

Mention emotion-laden encounters and incidents such as running into your divorced husband or ex-boyfriend with his latest. Mention any escalated frets or worries such as your son getting thrown into jail in Mexico, your daughter joining a religious cult. Report, too, on any upbeat events like getting a A in a college course in which you fully expected a C, or winning a contest. And be sure to keep watch on the Holmes and Rahe stress list in Chapter 3 and write down any of these significant life changes.

You might also be alert for those body signals of stress that we told you about in Chapter 3. Did you catch yourself clenching your fists or teeth, gripping the steering wheel until your knuckles were white?

**8. Diet.** Here you tell what meals and snacks you ate and at what hour of the day or night. Write down exactly what you ate and drank and the amounts or size of each portion (one half glass orange juice, two blueberry muffins, one strip bacon). Include cups of coffee and tea, all soft drinks, candy, gum, and any other little thing you slipped into your mouth. If you have a headache, note if the food or drink made you feel better or worse.

This is the most time-consuming and tedious part of the diary. Fortunately, if you are able to eliminate food and drink as headache causes in your case, you can eliminate this section, too.

**9. Activities and Exercise.** Here you give a rundown on what you did during the day and evening. How did you spend your time? Were you generally active or sedentary? Give just a quick overview on this, or even one sentence—a minute-by-minute rendition is unnecessary.

What you do want to spell out in depth are the particulars of your sports activities and exercise. Be specific about how many laps you swam, how many sets of tennis you played, how many holes of golf. Indicate the amount of time spent and how vigorous the exertion. For that much denigrated form of female exercise, housework, if it was unusually vigorous like waxing floors on your hands and knees, window cleaning, wall washing, etc., note this in your diary, too. In fact, include any out-of-the-ordinary physical activity. You will want to be able to see if exercise brings on or holds off a headache and if, when you have a headache, exercise relieves it or exacerbates it.

**10. Free-form Ranting.** Here is what may be the X-rated section of your journal. In this you let fly with fury, using whatever language you choose. You don't necessarily have to share this with your doctor or anyone else. This portion of your journal has a three-fold advantage. It has the salubrious effect of getting some of the festering anger out of your system—like pounding a pillow, and that is not a bad idea either. If you get those pent-up negative emotions out of your system and on paper then maybe they will stop popping out in the form of headaches. Then too, if you dump your complaints and wrath into your diary, maybe you won't have to dump them on your family and friends. (Take it from Barbara, constant headache dumping severely damages any human relationship be it personal or professional.)

It's also true that frequently in wrath as in wine there is truth. Your stream-of-consciousness outpouring just might give you some insight into the cause of your headaches that wouldn't be discoverable in the straight reportage of the rest of your diary.

Finally, it's possible you could turn out a new literary masterpiece. Self-revelations written in frank language are very big these days and your *Fear of Headaching* may top the bestseller list someday.

June's diary contained a free-form rant that might give you a glimmering of what you can do in this section of the diary. We wish we could present it to you in its original wild scrawl rather than in emotionless print. It would be a graphologist's delight.

Sunday, January 16, Laguna Beach
Awoke without headache. Restored bite plane after breakfast but still have bad sensations floating around bridge of nose.

Very morose and depressed all day with floating, odd sensations and extreme feeling of disorientation, as if someone had screwed an alien head onto my neck. Tried to get down to work, but ended up announcing to B. (Barbara) that I will never again go to another doctor for anything. I'm not afraid to die and am ready to die— indeed, *prefer* to die. I told B. I would truly like to go to her next (expletive deleted) miracle cure doctor and have him announce after the first time-consuming, expensive appointment, "(Expletive deleted), I don't have one (expletive deleted) idea of what is causing your (expletive deleted) headaches and I can't do a (expletive deleted) thing for you."

"Great!" I would say, "that's what I most wanted to hear from a doctor."

B. does not believe me, but I am giving up on the (expletive deleted) medical establishment. I can take care of my own diabetes and as for anything else, I prefer to die of it. An early death is a beautiful thing, especially if it is welcomed by the recipient.

Getting all this out of her system reduced the tensions that were starting to build up and June probably stopped clenching and grinding her teeth, because a short while later the feelings of disorientation and lightheadedness drifted away.

**11. Inner Communication (Optional).** If you find you take naturally to diary writing, as many women down through the literary ages have, then you may want to go further with it.

In her book, *The New Diary*, Tristine Rainer suggests numerous diary devices and techniques for self-analysis, including finding out the underlying causes of why you are afflicted with illness or pain.

The best *New Diary* device for our purposes is to write an imaginary dialogue with your head—or, better yet, with your headache—and let it reveal its message to you. As we mentioned before in discussing holism, illness is the body's unignorable way of telling you that you need to change your attitudes, your actions, or your reactions. Through a dialogue with your headache you may help yourself understand what changes you need to make.

To illustrate this kind of dialogue with a part of your body, we will use Ms. Rainer's example of a woman who had badly injured her right toe.

**Me**
Hey, right foot, what's all the trouble about?
**Right Foot**
Put your right foot forward.
**Me**
Are you trying to say that I have trouble getting ahead?
**Right Foot**
You got it.
**Me**
But what does that really mean?
**Right Foot**
It has to do with foresight. You step where you shouldn't, you leap without looking; you put your foot in it. You're careless.
**Me**
Gee, you're very reprimanding.
**Right Foot**
I'm a right foot.
**Me**
You sure are. Listen, I also have a left foot. It doesn't seem to give me trouble.
**Right Foot**
He's a follower. I'm a leader. You're having trouble with leadership. You're afraid to take a stand. You don't have a sure step.

**Me**
Well how am I supposed to get all those things?
**Right Foot**
Start thinking. Look and consider before you act. Slow down. Think carefully about your life. Plan carefully. You have no time for mistakes. I want to lead you in the right direction.
**Me**
That's all pretty clear. Will you heal now?
**Right Foot**
You bet. I'm good at that, though I'll be sore for awhile as a reminder.
**Me**
Aw, give me a break.
**Right Foot**
That's exactly what I'm doing.

Now that you have this example, you can move up to your headache and try having a conversation with it. Perhaps your headache will tell you that you're beating your head against a stone wall or that you've trapped your brain and are squeezing it to death and it wants out or that the mask you're wearing is too tight and you should take it off or, well, again, we don't want to structure you. You have to write *your* conversation with *your* head, because only in that way will you find the answer to the problem and a permanent cure for *your* headaches.

# PART TWO

## TREATING YOU AND YOUR HEADACHES: SOLVING THE MYSTERY

# 5

# TEMPORARY
# RELIEF MEASURES

$W$hile trying to do the investigation necessary to cure your headaches permanently — making your experiments and recording the results in your diary — you'll want some temporary relief. You'll need some holistic analgesics to give you respite from the acute stage of pain so that you can function well as a detective. After all, if Columbo or Miss Marple were confined to a room with someone continually zapping them over the head with a blackjack, they'd have a little trouble performing efficient detective work, too.

First, we want to give you some assurances about the risk of masking your pain with temporary relief measures. If there's something seriously wrong with you, is it dangerous to merely treat the symptom and ignore the cause? Not really, because in a sense Mother Nature protects you by not letting you wipe out the pain permanently. Whenever pain indicates a serious condition, it rears its (aching) head again and again and again.

This is why, in holistic thinking, pain is considered not an enemy to fight but a friend. Pain is trying to help you by making you aware that there are things going wrong somewhere in your body-mind-spirit-environment complex. It's letting you know you have to make some changes.

You may think that the headache itself is your only problem, that if there were some way to get rid of that wretched pain everything would be lovely. Not so. Take June's case again. Merely stopping the pain, as acupuncture did for a while, didn't solve her basic problems. Her bite was still misaligned, she was still putting herself under too much stress. Even if the headache had stayed away, something more serious and life-threatening would very likely have popped out later.

No, your friend pain is telling you something for your own good, maybe something you don't want to hear, but something that it is vitally important for you to listen to, understand, and act upon. And until you make the changes pain is telling you about, it will not keep quiet for long.

The techniques of relief from your nagging "friend" that we're going to include here are all holistic analgesics—they won't addict you or give you harmful side effects while they're helping you. We're covering massage, hand warming, acupuncture, acupressure, electro-acupuncture. Massage is particularly good for muscular headaches; hand warming is most helpful for vascular headaches; and acupuncture, acupressure, and electro-acupuncture work well for any kind of headache. Also, for those of you who feel you can't give up your drugs yet, we have some warnings and some advice about how to make them as effective and safe as possible.

Now let's see if we can stop that blackjack from hammering on your skull for a while.

# MASSAGE

Massage is an important holistic therapy for breaking up muscular tension and relieving pressure on the nerves. Doctors often send muscular-headache patients to professional masseuses (and masseurs) for deep-muscle massage. We heard an expert in rehabilitative medicine explain that, in order to work, the massage has to be deep enough to be painful. Chiropractors can also help muscular headache sufferers by manipulation, massage, and muscle stretching.

But here we want to give you some do-it-yourself home massage techniques that June found extremely relief-giving. We refer to what is called "zone therapy" or "reflexology," which is based on the theory that massaging certain areas of the hands and feet can relieve many physical problems. The technique works more or less the way that pressing certain acupuncture and acupressure points of the hands and feet (see Figures 3, 4, and 5 later on in this chapter) can ease pain in distant parts of the body like the head. Foot reflexology, as distinct from hand, is believed to be related to treatments in European sanatoriums where they send patients out to walk barefoot on the dewy grass.

Actually, our experience with massage came about when Barbara heard Dr. Joyce Brothers suggesting headache remedies on the radio one day. Included was the message that massage, especially of the hands and feet, could help reduce pain. The next time June had a headache Barbara tried massage on June's feet, which, incidentally were as cold as frozen fish fillets. She rubbed and kneaded June's toes, feet, ankles, and even calves for about half an hour until the fish fillets thawed and June began to feel the little breakings up of the headache, like snow beginning to melt, behind her nose. An hour later all the pain was gone. This headache buster didn't work every time for June, but it did frequently either break up the headache or at least diminish the intensity of the pain. Because of the change in foot temperature, we figured improving circulation could be, along with hitting acupressure points, possibly another headache-reducing benefit of the massage.

Since then, in order to understand this phenomenon better and improve in technique, we have researched the use of foot reflexology particularly for headaches. The best place to massage is the fleshy underpart of the big toes. Also, press each toe between the fingers until you locate the sore or tender places and massage these until the tenderness is gone.

If you do not have a willing and patient masseuse or masseur handy, you could try massaging your feet yourself, but we both feel that the relaxation and the being-cared-for and fussed-over qualities of having someone else do it are a good part of the therapy.

## HAND WARMING

There are two methods of warming the hands: by external means or through biofeedback. External hand warming is an old-wives'-tale remedy that is discounted by science, but many headache sufferers have told us they obtain some relief from it. You simply soak your hands in hot water, as hot as possible without burning your hands.

Two embellishments on this technique are to put cool compresses on your head or to put your feet in hot water. (Doing all three of these techniques at once would be a contortionist's delight.)

A doctor told us that external hand warming with hot water does not deliver the pain relief of the biofeedback type, which comes from within (see Chapter 7). Admittedly, hand warming with your mind is a more holistic method but it takes a lot more training than putting your hands in hot water does.

## ACUPUNCTURE

When June first considered having acupuncture treatments, we both had a few odd—and wrong—theories about how it works. We thought, as do many others, that the needles blocked the pain impulses. From some reading we did later, we learned that a more accepted theory states just the opposite.

According to this theory, acupuncture is not a blocking, but rather an unblocking. Throughout the body there runs an energy network composed of channels that the Chinese call meridians. Along each of these meridians are located many acupuncture points (there are hundreds of these). When a needle is stuck into an acupuncture point it stimulates the flow of energy which then proceeds to course throughout the body, restoring the energy balance and curing what ails you.

An even newer theory is that acupuncture stimulates the nervous system to secrete its own painkillers, called endorphins, a Greek word meaning "the morphine within." Endorphins are chemically similar to compounds found in opium and their effect appears to be similar to that of morphine.

Theory aside, does acupuncture hurt? Dr. C. Norman Shealy, director of the Pain Rehabilitation Center in La Crosse, Wisconsin, says, "Needle acupuncture in itself is painful, although the Chinese and many others have given the impression that acupuncture does not hurt." He attributes the does-it-or-doesn't-it-hurt confusion to semantics, explaining that, while we have only one word for pain, the Chinese have dozens. The word they apply to the sensation of an acupuncture needle hurting is "sour."

As you remember from June's experience, it *does* hurt. June found quite a bit of pain with about one third of the fifty needle insertions in each treatment and experienced additional discomfort from the electrical current attachments that sent a strong vibration through the needles.

But despite the pain, acupuncture did keep June headache-free for months. And she is not alone in her success with acupuncture. Many others have experienced varying degrees of relief because of it. We even saw a bumper sticker that read, "I have been helped by acupuncture." A friend also told us that she was talking about acupuncture and headaches with a neurosurgeon who is a resident at Hong Kong's British Hospital, where, as the doctor explained, it is illegal to do acupuncture. What does he himself do when he has a headache? He carries a needle in his pocket and gives himself an acupuncture treatment.

Acupuncture does not have to be such a painful experience. Not all acupuncturists stick in fifty needles for headaches; many use far fewer. Besides this, we later found out that the doctor June went to was not universally considered one of the best. In fact, his prices were out of line, and he seemed to specialize in sticking staples into people's earlobes to help them "instantly" lose weight or stop smoking. If you shop more carefully for an acupuncturist and look over the setup with a more suspicious eye than June did, you are likely to have better, less expensive, and more humane treatment.

To make an unscientific generalization, we've found in talking to people who've had acupuncture that those who are most pleased with the treatments and results are those who've had Oriental therapists. This may be because these acupuncturists have had lifelong, in-depth experience with acupuncture, while sometimes the Westerners have had only a relatively thin layer of acupuncture training on top of their standard medical education.

Fortunately, the law (at least in California) now allows acupuncturists without medical degrees to treat patients if they work under the direct supervision of M.D.s. Therefore, more and more professional acupuncturists are coming onto the scene. Unfortunately, so are a number of illegal practitioners, but since some of these have a reputation for being Hepatitis Harrys, we couldn't recommend them.

If you find that there is no legal acupuncturist in your area or if the idea of the needles and pain and cost is too much for you, then there is another way of energy-flowing your pain away.

## ACUPRESSURE

Acupressure, pressing the acupuncture points with the fingers instead of using needles, has the tremendous advantage that for the most part you can do it yourself on yourself and it's free. All the equipment you need is already there, literally at your fingertips.

Possibly one of the reasons acupuncture has a much better press than acupressure in this country is that we're very much a tool-oriented culture. Many doctors seem to rely on instruments and seldom perform any of the old-fashioned laying on of hands. We've all become conditioned to think that an instrument improves the treatment.

In order to learn firsthand about acupressure, Barbara took a course in it at Valley College where we work. When she told her instructor that she wanted to learn the pressure points for headaches, the instructor, before giving this information, made it very clear that "there are no pressure points for headaches caused by a bad marriage or by eating all your meals at fast food franchises or by never exercising." Still, there are headache points, and acupressure may prove to be effective digital aspirin for you.

Just as in aspirin, in acupressure you have more than one brand to choose from. Among the several methods there is *G-Jo*, a Chinese term that can be loosely translated as "first aid." There is *shiatzu*, meaning "finger pressure" in Japanese. There is also the Touch for Health method developed by a chiropractor, John F. Thie. Each method has its unique characteristics, but they all share many of the same basic principles and most of the same pressure points, the same points used for acupuncture relief of headaches.

Adherents to all methods of acupressure agree that you should use it for preventing a headache, as well as for relieving the pain when you already have one. If you do the treatments regularly on a daily basis, whether you have a headache or not, you may be able to make your headaches fewer, farther between, and less severe.

The best way to learn acupressure would be to learn it directly from an acupressurist, either in private sessions or in a class, such as those being given at community colleges and in university extension programs. However, many headache sufferers can help themselves by using acupressure points they have only read about. Let us press on and see if you are one of those.

If you have long fingernails, please clip them off your thumbs and file them down so that you aren't in danger of puncturing yourself if you press your thumb ends and nails very hard into your vulnerable flesh. For acupressure to work it has to hurt somewhat, but you shouldn't wound yourself.

Some experienced acupressurists work with their fingertips rather than their thumbs, but we find it easier to manage the recommended 20 pounds of pressure with the better angle of attack and greater strength that the thumbs provide. Incidentally, that 20 pounds is a lot of pressure. In order to know just how much, you should experiment by pressing your thumb on a bathroom scale. June tried this and claims her thumbs are too weak to push that hard. Our advice, then, is to settle for pressing as hard as you can. Just make sure that you always press the points on both sides of the body, since your objective is to restore balance.

When you're trying to locate an acupressure point, probe hard around the area until you feel a tender spot or the dramatic reverberating shock sensation similar to the one you feel when you bang your elbow. It feels as if you've hit a nerve because, in fact, you have. Finding points often takes quite a bit of probing. Don't get discouraged.

The first two points we're going to explain to you are the classic headache points, *ho-ku* and *feng-chih*. To find *ho-ku* (shown in Fig. 3) hold your left hand in front of you so that you are seeing the top or backside of it. Stretch your thumb out at a right angle to the hand so that it forms an L with the index finger. Take your right thumb and run it down your left index finger past the knuckle down to where the finger bone is connected to the thumb bone. This is just behind the webbing that runs between the thumb and index finger. Bend your right thumb at the first joint and start probing—hard—with your right thumbnail along the bone (*not* the tendon) in your hand (*not* your thumb bone) until you get that hit-nerve feeling. When you do, you have found *ho-ku*. Press on this point with your 20 pounds of pressure for about thirty seconds.

Now find *ho-ku* the same way on your right hand and press it.

To find the second basic headache point, *feng-chih* (shown in Fig. 4), drop your chin to your chest. Feel the back of your neck to locate the two indentations at the base of your skull and probe upward against the skull bone until you locate the tender or "elbow-bang" spots. When you do, give them the 20 pounds of pressure for thirty seconds. If you can't find the points, just massage this area hard. You can press or massage both sides simultaneously, if you like.

June found that when the acupressure was starting to work she felt a coolness in the headache pain area. Others report a kind of decongesting feeling in the pain center. Your sensations may be different still. Monitor your feelings carefully for any sign that means the acupressure is touching your pain. This will be a signal that you should work seriously with acupressure. Of course, if it relieves

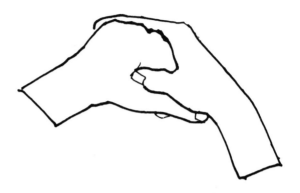

Figure 3

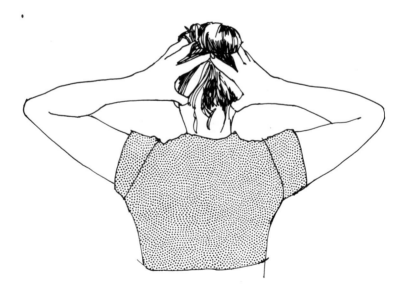

Figure 4

your pain entirely, we know we won't have to tell you to work seriously with it.

Working seriously means acquainting yourself with and using the other points related to headaches in the same way as with *ho-ku* and *feng-chih*. Fig. 5 shows you their names and locations.

Now for the "buts" about acupressure. Many people, ourselves included, sometimes find it difficult to locate the points. For example, once when Barbara was trying to find *tai-yang*, an elusive point located one fingerbreadth away from the outer bone of the eyesocket and just before the temple indentation, it took her about a half hour of probing and drawing lines with an eyebrow pencil. It was enough to *give* her a muscle-tension headache. And to tell the truth, she never was positive she found it.

It's also sometimes tiring, if not impossible, to apply 20 pounds of pressure for the required thirty seconds on several successive points, especially if you have a headache at the time. Not only that, but the pressure even for that brief period is uncomfortable and sometimes produces bruises.

If you experience any or all of these problems with acupressure, don't despair. There is an easy and, all things considered, relatively inexpensive solution for you. And it is a new advance in headache treatment that is gaining recognition by doctors.

## ELECTROACUPUNCTURE

Technically, this is known as transcutaneous neurological stimulation, but since that's something of a tongue twister to say and a mind twister to contemplate, we call it by its shorter descriptor, electroacupuncture.

It combines the ancient Chinese wisdom of acupuncture with modern Western scientific advances. It gives you a headache treatment that is as effective as the most skilled acupuncture yet *does not hurt at all* and, what's more, you

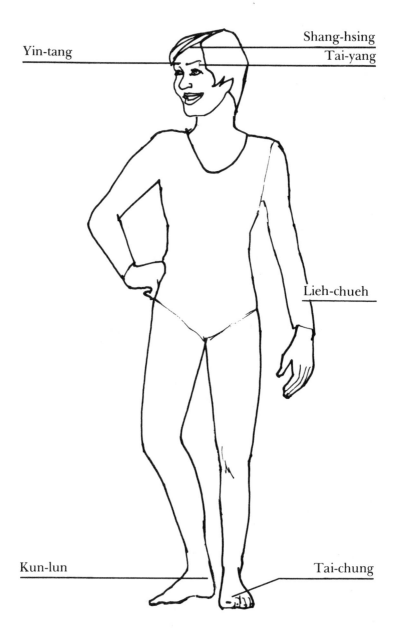

Yin-tang

Shang-hsing
Tai-yang

Lieh-chueh

Kun-lun

Tai-chung

Figure 5

can do it yourself on yourself at home with a minimum of instruction. It doesn't take the kind of finger or thumb strength that acupressure does and you can always find each point quickly, easily, and surely.

All these seemingly magical processes are performed by a small mechanism, the TNS Point and Rolectric Massage Stimulator, called the Rolectric Massage for short. As you can see in Fig. 6, it is about the same size and shape as an electric razor and is powered by a standard 9 volt battery. The cost is under $200, and is covered by your health insurance if your doctor recommends its use. Even Medicare financially acknowledges its merits as a therapeutic device.

How did this electroacupuncture instrument come into being and why is this the first time you've heard about it? It has only been available since 1976 and is the culmination of years of experimentation and research by Dr. Charles Ledergerber, a gynecologist, who is a Fellow of both the American College of Surgeons and the American College of Gynecologists as well as a Diplomate of the American Board of Gynecology and Obstetrics.

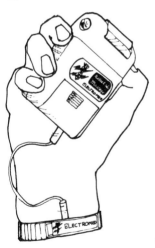

Figure 6

Dr. Ledergerber wanted to find a way to relieve pain without using drugs, which always have detrimental side effects. Acupuncture to him seemed to be the logical choice, so he studied it intensively in China, Russia, and France. Combining all this research with his previous studies of Western medical experiments in the application of electrical energy to change nervous system function, Dr. Ledergerber created the Rolectric Massage for the treatment of chronic pain. The actual engineering was done by one of the inventors of the laser beam.

Dr. Ledergerber's dedication to finding drug-free pain relief was not only for his patients. He was also motivated by his wife, a victim of a painful form of arthritis that destroys the cartilage in the hip bone. Mrs. Ledergerber was helped by electroacupuncture and now instead of being bedridden is relatively pain-free and is able to walk with crutches and work as a therapist. She was in a sense one of the developers of the Rolectric Massage, because as the subject of her husband's experiments, she helped Dr. Ledergerber test which frequencies were the most effective, which acupuncture points worked best, and so on.

Now Mrs. Ledergerber uses the Rolectric Massage to help sufferers of all kinds. A trained psychotherapist from Johns Hopkins, she is a pain therapist who combines electroacupuncture and psychological counseling in her treatments. In a one-year follow-up study of thirty of her headache patients, all but five had received some measure of relief.

Mrs. Ledergerber's basic routine in treating headaches is as follows: First, she checks out one acupuncture point in the area of the pain with a point finder. This is a small electronic stylus-like device that is used in the office to gauge the electrical charge coming from the point. If there is an organic reason for the pain (that is, if it is physiological rather than psychological), the point on the side of the body where the pain is shows a decreased electric resistance compared to the corresponding point on the other side.

She then takes the Rolectric Massage and gives the patient a general relaxation and well-being treatment. It is her belief that many people would not have pain if they could just relax. She works both with the roller electrode part of the instrument, which she moves over the skin surface in much the same way as if she were using an electric razor, and with the ball electrode, which she touches to the appropriate acupuncture relaxation points. The Rolectric Massage has several adjustments so you can get exactly the stimulation strength you need—the strength that you are able to feel but isn't at all uncomfortable.

She then goes on to the special headache points we mentioned in the acupressure section: *ho-ku*, *feng-chih*, and several others. She touches each point on each side of the body for approximately thirty seconds.

When she is finished, if all has gone well the headache is relieved, and when she checks the original point with her point finder, the charges have been equalized and the body's electricity has been balanced again.

When she demonstrated the Rolectric Massage on us, we were fascinated—and amazed. Since we'd both struggled to find the points when we were working with acupressure, it was stunning to move the little ball electrode over the area of the *ho-ku* point and have it zing when the point was hit and send tingles up the index finger.

Like acupressure, electroacupuncture works best if it is done regularly on a daily basis, perhaps as part of a morning routine. A treatment takes only a few minutes if you just do the major headache points, but its effect normally lasts up to twenty-four hours.

The only people who should not use electroacupuncture are epileptics, pregnant women, and those who wear pacemakers. Naturally you should not use it to try to permanently alleviate a pain of unknown origin rather than going to a doctor to find the organic cause of the condition.

Mrs. Ledergerber would also be the first to admit that, especially for those with headaches, life and attitudinal changes are necessary for a cure. Still, electroacupuncture can break the headache pattern for many sufferers.

The Rolectric Massage can be ordered by mail, so even if you live somewhere in the wilderness you can still obtain one. For those who cannot come into the office for treatment or instruction in the use of the Rolectric Massage, Mrs. Ledergerber has prepared an instruction sheet, but if you are still confused you can telephone her and she'll try to clarify.

There are some other electroacupuncture machines coming onto the market, but none of those that we've heard of has either the ball electrode or the rolling-over-the-pain feature of the Rolectric Massage. Also the other machines work on AC. The Rolectric Massage works on DC because Dr. Ledergerber discovered that, since the body itself is DC, using the same kind of current is more effective.

As of this writing, the Rolectric Massage costs $185, but inflation being what it is, the price may inevitably rise. The price strikes us as eminently reasonable, especially when you consider that it's less than what it would have cost June for only four sessions with her acupuncturist.

For further information, write Electromed Incorporated, 9400 Brighton Way, Suite 410, Beverly Hills, CA 90210. Phone: (213) 274-8582; (213) 274-8338.

## DRUGS

In order to get some kind of relief many women, with or without the cooperation and assistance of a doctor, try to knock out their headache pain with pills or get themselves zonked to the point that they're oblivious to any feeling.

We have become what you might call drug resistors, especially since so many of them did so little for June's condition. Drugs may work for acute, short-lived pain, but for the chronic pain we're involved with here, they have the dual problem of quickly losing their effectiveness and of causing addiction. On top of these negatives, they can have harmful to disastrous side effects, especially when they interact with other drugs. In short, your headaches can't kill you, but the drugs you take to relieve them can.

Our main objection to using painkillers, tranquilizers, mood elevators, antidepressants, antihistamines, and all the rest of the chemical crutches many sufferers lean on is that drugs do not heal. They can at best only help the body do its own healing. At worst, they can prevent the body from healing itself.

Still, we acknowledge that many of you take drugs of one kind or another for interim survival purposes, so we'd like to pass on to you a few tips from June's headache drug days.

Stoic that she tried to be, June would often hold off taking the drug as long as possible, finally giving in when the pain became too intense to bear. This, she later discovered, was dead wrong. Even with aspirin, and certainly with something like Cafergot, to get any kind of relief you have to hit the headache while it's still weak and tentative. If you wait until it grows into a monster its hide becomes too tough for a drug to penetrate. If you know from experience that you're going to wind up taking the drug anyway, then take it at the first twinge.

After brief experiments with Darvon, Fiorinal, codeine, and other painkillers of high repute among doctors, June came to the conclusion that she personally couldn't beat that old standby, aspirin. And if taken with a cup of coffee, it works even better for vascular headaches than if taken alone, because the caffeine in coffee constricts swollen blood vessels. We found out that a Mayo Clinic study comparing aspirin with codeine, Darvon, Talwin, and acetaminophen and phenacetin (these last two are contained in A.P.C., Empirin Compound, Excedrin, Fabrinol, Nebs, Percogesic, Tempra, and Tylenol) showed that "among all analgesics and narcotics available for oral use, none have been demonstrated to show a consistent advantage over aspirin for the relief of any type of pain." The dosage of aspirin used in this study was 650 mg.

The chart below is the FDA's recommendation for limiting aspirin tablets. As you see, tablets come in different strengths, so be sure to read your bottle label to know precisely what you are taking.

### Recommended Adult Dosage Schedule for Nonstandard Aspirin Tablets

| Aspirin per Tablet | Initial Dosage | Subsequent Dosage and Schedule | Maximum 24-Hour Dosage |
|---|---|---|---|
| 400 milligrams (6.15 grains) | 1 to 2 | 1 after 3 hours | 9 |
| 421 milligrams (6.48 grains) | 1 to 2 | 1 after 3 hours | 9 |
| 4.85 milligrams (7.46 grains) | 1 to 2 | 1 after 4 hours or 2 after 6 hours | 8 |
| 500 milligrams (7.69 grains) | 1 to 2 | 1 after 3 hours or 2 after 6 hours | 8 |
| 650 milligrams (10) grains) | 1 | 1 after 4 hours | 6 |

For your aspirin to remain effective you should protect it by *not* keeping it in the bathroom. Those two basics of the bathroom atmosphere—heat and humidity—are the worst enemies of all drugs, but especially of aspirin. The medicine cabinet doesn't protect them, neither do the "airtight" bottles. Since the kitchen is usually as bad as the bathroom for heat and humidity, the bedroom is probably the best place to keep all of your drugs.

And now a word of caution about aspirin dosage. Aspirin irritates the lining of the stomach and if you have ulcers or a tendency toward indigestion you may want to stay away from it, especially in dosages of over five tablets a day. You can sidestep aspirin's irritating effect somewhat by always drinking a *full* glass of water with it. Even better, chew it up mixed with a mouthful of milk or pulverize it and mix it in a glass of milk. And if you are taking high dosages of vitamin C you ought to be aware that this vitamin prolongs and intensifies the effect of aspirin in the body and may enhance its irritating effects. Alcohol is another aspirin irritation enhancer.

## Drug Interactions

The problems of drug side effects and interactions are more complex and will force you to do some studying and research on drugs you're using. Joe Graedon, author of *The People's Pharmacy*, calls drug interactions "the Achilles' heel of the medical profession." He likens mixing drugs to playing Russian roulette because "you never know when a particular combination will produce a lethal outcome."

Although one drug can diminish or even wipe out another drug's effectiveness, more often what happens is *potentiation*. Each drug augments the effect of the other. This can be by far a greater problem than lack of effectiveness. You may have heard the story of radio commentator Dorothy Kilgallen, who came home from work one evening and had one or two drinks. They reacted in an adverse potentiated manner with a prescription drug she'd been taking and caused her death. Although hers is a particularly well-publicized occurrence, it is not an uncommon one.

It would be lovely if doctors had the time to carefully ascertain what drugs you're taking before prescribing another. They generally don't. You can help them—and yourself—by keeping a list of the drugs you already take and by asking your doctor *pointedly* if there would be any problems with the new one.

Some pharmacies are now keeping a record of every prescription issued to a patient. They check and warn you if you're running any interaction risk. The difficulty with this is twofold: First, you don't always buy your drugs at the same pharmacy, especially if you're comparison shopping; and second, not all drugs you can get in trouble with are prescription drugs, for example, aspirin, alcohol, and vitamins.

What to do? Even though drugs are a nonholistic treatment, if you do take them you should at least adhere to the holistic principle of taking the responsibility for what they do to you. Read all about the drugs you're taking in Joe Graedon's excellent and easy-to-understand *The People's Pharmacy*. Give particular attention to the section on drug interactions.

If you have a tolerance for fine print and medical terminolgy follow this up with a visit to the library and check out your drugs in the *Physician's Desk Reference (PDR)*. This volume tells all there is to know about individual drugs and their actions, reactions, and side effects. The main information for a drug is listed under the name of the company that produces it. To find the name of the company, look up the drug in the front of the book. If you still have trouble finding the entry for the drug, ask the librarian for help. That's what they're there for. (Believe us. We know.)

When you find the correct entry read everything there on the subject of the drug you're taking. It may make you a hypochondriac, but that's better than making you nonexistent.

In the final drug analysis, we think Joe Graedon makes

two points that are especially important for you to remember.

1. Try to avoid taking more than one drug at a time. When that becomes impossible, monitor your own system's reactivity and sensitivity. At the first sign of trouble, head straight for your doctor's office. Better yet, use the phone.
2. There is no such thing as a 100 percent safe drug.

**Marijuana**

We will finish off this section on drugs with an illusory headache relief measure that you may at some time in your long headache career have been—or will be—tempted to try.

June was in one of her usual desperate periods. She'd had a headache for over a week. She had to find something, *anything* to get rid of it. The something, *anything* that she came up with was marijuana. She knew of a woman who had suffered excruciating back pains that were relieved after she went to a pot party. But it didn't work for June. If anything, her headache got a little worse, probably from the smoke, which had always been a headache activator for her.

We've read that the first few times you sample marijuana you often don't get any reaction, especially if you've had a nodding acquaintance with alcohol. You've developed a cross-tolerance, meaning you've reached the point that it takes more alcohol to get an effect and the first time you smoke marijuana, you need more than most beginners would to feel its effects. With more crossness than tolerance, June gave up marijuana.

Dr. Lee Kudrow in an article in the *National Migraine Foundation Newsletter* reported on a marijuana study conducted at the California Medical Clinic for Headache. This study was of twenty headache patients (their average age was 22) who admitted smoking marijuana. When asked what effect smoking marijuana during the early stages of a headache had on the headache, 40 percent said it made no change, 40 percent said it aborted the headache, and 20 percent said it made the headache worse. In the later stages of the headache, the marijuana caused no change in 35 percent of the patients, aborted or improved the headache in 5 percent, and made it worse in 60 percent.

As for marijuana smoking making headaches worse, that's not the end of it. One headache specialist reported a case in which a 12-year-old boy was sent to him for headache treatment. It turned out that the marijuana he was sneaking at school was *causing* his headaches.

Considering these negatives and all of the continuing unknowns and illegalities of marijuana, it seems to us that for headache relief there are better methods.

# 6

## RELAXATION AND EXERCISE THERAPIES FOR THE BODY

A policeman arrests the criminal after the crime has already been committed. A sociologist, on the other hand, tries to discover and rectify the underlying problems that turn people into criminals and thus tries to prevent the crime altogether. When it comes to disease, our Western medicine plays the cop role, trying to arrest the disease after it strikes. Western medicine concentrates on *sickness*. Eastern or holistic medicine is the sociologist working in the area of crime prevention, trying to change the conditions that lead to the disease. The emphasis is on *wellness*.

No matter how far from—or close to—the solution of your headache mystery you are, it's time you played the sociologist and put forth some effort toward headache prevention. Keep in mind the aphorism of the ancient yoga philosopher, Patanjali: "Pain which has not yet come is avoidable."

We are going to show you the two routes to take simultaneously toward the avoidance of pain. Researchers at the

119

Menninger Foundation have proven scientifically what holism knows experientially: Every change in the body produces a change in the mind; every change in the mind produces a change in the body. Relaxation and physical exercise therapies unclench your mental fist; stress-reducing techniques of the mind create a tension-free body; and both combine to set up a barrier against attacks from disease and pain.

This chapter takes you along the body-to-mind route via progressive relaxation, stretching, and the most popular aerobic exercise, running. The following chapter will take you from the mind to the body by the stress-reducing vehicles of autogenic training, meditation, biofeedback, and guided imagery.

## R<sub>X</sub>ERCISE

A major problem with many headache sufferers, especially women headache sufferers, is that they're hypokinetic. That is to say, they're underexercised. Dr. Heuser, speaking to doctors at a UCLA headache seminar, pointed out that certain chemical changes that take place in the body during headaches are the reverse of the changes that take place in the body during exercise. He spoke in terms of levels of beta hydroxylase and monoamine oxidase, but, as he added, "If you can get the patient to exercise, you can forget a lot of the chemistry." Some headache doctors consider exercise so important that they have added medical exercise experts to their staffs and have set aside a special room for exercise therapy.

There are actually two categories of physical activity for you to consider in your headache prevention program: muscular exercises and aerobic exercises. Muscular exercises are of course most effective for those of you whose headaches are muscular in origin. Aerobic exercises build up your cardiovascular system and consequently are especially recommended for those of you who suffer from vascular headaches. But since it's not always possible to decide which kind of headache you have or, indeed, if both muscles and blood vessels contribute to your problem, just to be on the safe side it might be wise to incorporate both into your program.

## MUSCULAR EXERCISES

### Progressive Relaxation

Exercise therapist Linda Sharp says one of her greatest challenges is getting headache patients to know what a relaxed muscle even feels like. Many of them have been so tense for so long that they consider muscular tension to be their natural state. The following exercises are for those of you who can't tell a tense muscle from a relaxed one.

Progressive relaxation, or deep muscle relaxation, as it's sometimes called, is a system of first tensing a part of the body and then untensing it in order to feel the difference and thereby become capable of making the transition from tension to relaxation yourself. It was developed over fifty years ago by a Chicago physician, Edmund Jacobson.

Dr. Jacobson based his method on laboratory experiments that proved that when your muscles are completely relaxed, so are your mind and your emotions. He also did experiments showing that the sensation of pain is less intense or even not felt at all if muscles are relaxed. And what are relaxed muscles? They are muscles that are totally limp. You are neither contracting (tightening) them nor holding them rigid.

Progressive relaxation is a very easy technique to learn, but it does take patience. It takes most people two or three weeks to learn the techniques if they practice half an hour a day five days a week. You can hire a therapist who specializes in "Jacobsonian therapy," you can buy mail-order tapes to use at home, or you can learn to do it yourself by reading our directions here.

The training program depends, first, on repetition—

that is, *daily* pratice—and, second, effortlessness—that is, the less conscious effort you bring to untensing the muscles, the more relaxation you attain. It's the old Bauhaus architectural dictum of "less is more."

In the learning sessions, you experience over and over again the difference of sensation between extremely tense and extremely relaxed muscles until you recognize the difference without any doubt or hesitation. Once you know exactly what your muscles are doing, not only can you control your tendency to tense up but you become aware of when you are locking some part of yourself into one of those stiff and awkward postures that can cause headaches.

Now let's go through a practice session of progressive relaxation. You may want to have someone read this to you at first or, if you have a tape recorder, you may want to record it and listen to yourself tell yourself what to do. The value of this entire procedure is to plunge you into tension and then have the tension dissolve as you let go. You really only have to *think* about tightening a body part to engage the muscles, but in this practice session we're exaggerating to illustrate the contrast between tight and loose. Work slowly. Hold each tension position for twenty to thirty seconds. Don't rush.

> Sit in a high-backed chair or lie on your back on a carpeted floor or mat. Take a deep breath and hold it a moment. Breathe through your nostrils and breathe from the abdomen if you can. As you exhale slowly, try to let go of tension. Keep up a rhythmical pattern of breathing for a couple of minutes.
>
> Direct your attention to your right hand. (If you are left-handed, start with your left hand and revise the following instructions accordingly.) Clench your fist tightly. Observe your forearm; see it become tight, too. Hold. Stretch your fingers out and allow yourself to relax again after twenty or thirty seconds of tension. Be aware of what is

happening to your muscles, but don't be judgmental.

Make another tight fist with your right hand. Be aware of your muscles all the way up to your elbow. Hold. Let go slowly. Sense the difference between tenseness and relaxation.

Now direct your attention to your left hand and make a tight fist. Notice how your arm feels. Hold. Slowly let go. Next, with your right hand push down on your chair or the floor. Sense how your upper arm tightens. Hold. Relax and feel the flow of energy leaving. Now push with your left hand, hold, and then let go.

Hunch your shoulders so that you feel tension in your shoulders and in the back of your neck. Make it extreme. Hold. Then float down. Let your shoulders fall. Sense the muscles tense and then feel them relax.

With your hands, arms, and shoulders relaxed, push the back of your head hard against the chair or the floor. Sense the tension in the back of the neck. Hold. Then relax and let your head float.

Now the chin. Tighten it. Clench your teeth. Hold. Then relax and allow your mouth to open a bit. Be slack-jawed.

Push your tongue against the roof of your mouth. Hard. Hold. Then allow it to flop down. Notice how it seems to get larger as it relaxes.

Tighten your eyes. The purse-string muscles go around them. Close the purse. Hold. Allow your eyes to relax slowly.

Frown. Make a deep above-the-nose crease. Slowly relax. Do this particular exercise three times.

Next raise your eyebrows all the way up. Hold until you get the feel, then lower.

The scalp muscle runs from the edge of the hair line to the back of the head. If you push your eyebrows, your ears, and the back of your head upward, you will be contracting your scalp muscles. Hold. Now let down.

Tighten the muscles below the shoulders by arching your back. Hold. Then relax.

Next tighten the abdomen—make it hard. Hold, and then slowly let go.

The final step is to tighten your legs and feet. Stiffen your right leg. Hold. Relax it. Make your left leg rigid, hold, and then let the muscles smooth out. Study the feel of long, stretched-out, expanded leg muscles. Curl the toes of your right foot—make a fist of your foot. Hold. Then let go. Do the same with the left foot. Tighten, hold, release.

You will feel totally released from all tension—muscular or otherwise—at the end of your progressive relaxation practice session. You will feel good all over. The more you practice, the deeper your relaxation.

For headache sufferers it's a good idea to give the muscles of the eyes, head, and neck special relaxation treatments, maybe in the middle of the day or at night. Begin with the shoulder hunch and work your way through the tense-untense sequence up to and including the scalp muscles.

As you gain skill you can streamline your sessions and relax without first tensing. Just quickly check the different muscles mentally, then relax them physically.

The final stage of deep muscle relaxation is to relax all of your body at the same time. Check for feedback from different muscles and relax any that feel tense. Finally, you should be able to relax all over in only twenty seconds or, if you get to be championship caliber, in only five seconds. Jacobson's goal with his patients was to teach them to relax muscles as quickly as they could contract them.

One last dividend you can expect if you master the skill of deep muscle relaxation is a soft, youthful face. A furrowed brow, tight eye muscles, hardened cheek and lip muscles, a clenched jaw—all this leads to a haggard expression on a wrinkled one-hundred-year-old-woman face. So if you want to change face, turn to Jacobson before you have to turn to Elizabeth Arden.

If you seem to have a natural affinity for this method of treatment, you can send for an intensive professional course composed of three cassettes. They're available from Instructional Dynamics, Inc., 450 East Ohio Sreet, Chicago, IL 60611. The cost is about $30 including shipping. The program is called "Daily Living with Tensions and Anxieties, Relaxation Exercises I, II, and III." The recording is by Dr. Arnold A. Lazarus. We found Dr. Lazarus' accent rather distracting and the pace very, very slow, but this may be just the kind of approach that works for you.

Another commercial cassette is "Program for Learning Deep Muscle Relaxation" by John Marquis, Ph.D. This one is $10 and can be purchased from Self-Management Schools, 745 Distel Dr., Los Altos, CA 94122. It comes with an eleven-page explanation and direction sheet that is exceedingly helpful. Dr. Marquis considers the tape excellent for ridding yourself of muscle-tension headaches. The second half of his tape is devoted entirely to eye and throat muscles because those areas of the body get messages from the brain to tighten up when too many thoughts and images are whirling around under your skull. If you relax these muscles, you diminish this overactivity, get mentally relaxed, and minimize the chances of getting a headache.

### Stretching Exercises

Some books on headaches and many exercise therapy and yoga books recommend certain physical exercises for relieving headaches, but we think of them more as preventive measures. Eye, face, neck, shoulder, and back exercises can reduce muscular tensions and stretch those shortened muscles that may trigger headaches. In fact, June realizes that if she had practiced the exercises we're going to describe here on a regular basis—say three times a day every day—she might have avoided a lot of headaches. Now, older and wiser, when she feels herself getting tight in her eyes, jaws, neck, shoulders, or back, she stops and does some of these muscle stretchers and relaxers. They *do*

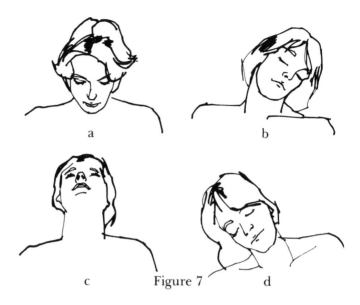

a
b
c Figure 7 d

help because they keep you from tying your muscular kinks into Gordian knots that no headache sufferer could possibly cut by herself.

When doing these exercises try to develop a sense of body awareness. As yoga instructors advise, turn off your ordinary mind, the one that's forever churning like a washing machine. Move slowly, smoothly into the stretch. *Be* the stretch. Experience it mentally as well as physically. Breathe deeply from the abdomen—the stomach should go out during inhalation and in during exhalation. (Place your hand on your abdomen to make sure your breathing is correct.) As you breathe, try to feel as if you are actually breathing into the muscle you're stretching.

**Head Rolls.** These are sometimes called neck rolls, because the neck is the part of you that gets the workout. You simply drop your head forward with your chin close to your chest and then you slowly roll your head in a complete circle first to the left and then to the right, as in Fig. 7. It's very important to roll slowly. A good technique is to pause several seconds when you get to your shoul-

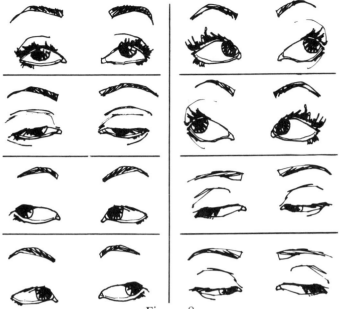

Figure 8

der, then pause again when your head is hanging backward and again over your other shoulder.

The more snap, crackle, and pop you hear when you do this exercise, the more good it's doing you. When June first did head rolls, she heard a kind of pizzicato string-snapping quartet each time she rolled. Now, since she's a regular yoga exercise disciple (head rolls are a yoga exercise), she hears only an occasional bit of cracking.

You should be able, after you loosen up, to do at least five head rolls. If they are too much for you at first, just drop your head forward and then drop it backward to stretch the throat. Hold several seconds in each position. Even this simple maneuver is very relaxing.

**Eye Circles.** Eye circles can be done almost anytime, anywhere. You probably never thought of exercising your eye muscles, but it's a very relaxing and refreshing thing to do—headaches or no headaches.

Fig. 8 illustrates this exercise. Holding your head level

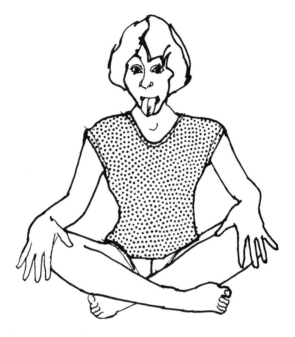

Figure 9

all the time, first look toward the ceiling, then drop your eyes toward the floor, then to the extreme right and then to the extreme left. Next, swing your eyes to the upper left corner, then down diagonally to the lower right corner, then to the upper right and down to the left. Again, don't move too quickly; hold each position a few seconds to keep yourself in a relaxing rhythm. And finally, just move your eyes in a continuous circle first to the left and then to the right. Do this exercise about three times.

**The Yoga Lion.** The yoga lion position is definitely not for public performance, and you will see why the first time you do this exercise.

Sit on the floor in a cross-legged position. In the classic yoga lion you push your head forward, but we recommend keeping your head in a normal position because the

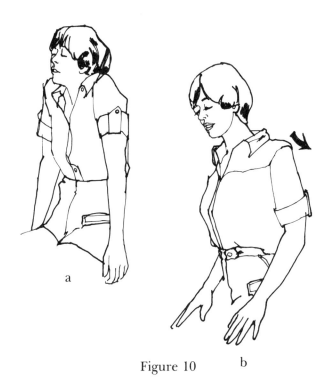

Figure 10    b

head-forward position is risky for headache sufferers since it can trigger headaches for some women (see Postural Swords in Chapter 3). Stick out your tongue as far as you can and open your eyes as wide as you can. Either rest your hands on your knees or, in the more classic manner, stretch your fingers wide apart as if you were a lion extending its claws. You should look somewhat like the woman in Fig. 9. Hold this pose for at least a slow count of ten. This drains the blood from the face and relaxes it.

**Shoulder Rolls.** For these you stand or sit with your arms hanging loose at your sides. As in Figure 10, hunch your shoulders toward your ears until your neck is sunk down between them (see Fig. 10a). Then roll your shoulders back and down until you are back to your beginning position (see Fig. 10b). These movements should

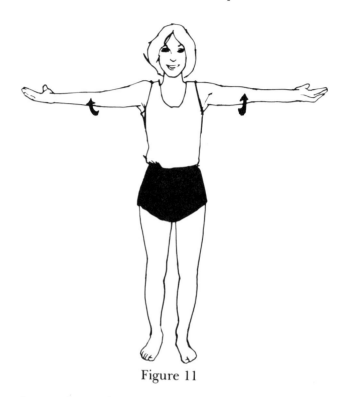

Figure 11

be slow and continuous and there should be a lot of tightening as you go through them and a lot of loosening as you end each roll. Pause between rolls and experience the totally unclenched sensation you feel. Repeat ten times.

**Arm Circles.** Here is another one for tight shoulders. Lift your arms up and hold them level with your shoulders, palms up. Now move them in little circles while they're extended (see Fig. 11). You can go counter clockwise first about ten times and then turn the palms down and go clockwise about ten times.

**Chest Muscle Stretcher.** An orthopedist once told June that the muscles at the back of her shoulders were sore a lot because the muscles in front were weak. After all, muscles work in pairs. He advised her to work on the upper

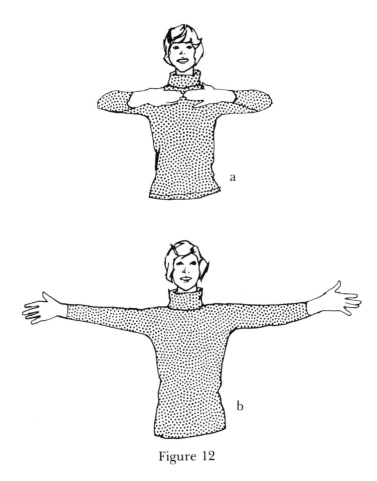

Figure 12

chest muscles to relieve the pain in the back. A good way to do this is to raise your arms to shoulder level and bend them across the chest until the fingertips touch (see Fig. 12a). Now open your arms out again (see Fig. 12b). Repeat the opening and closing movement ten or twelve times, pushing out with a strong thrust.

**Neck and Upper Back Stretch.** Lie down on the floor. Put your feet flat on the floor and your knees up together. Clasp your hands behind your head and slowly pull your head, neck, and shoulders up and forward, feeling the

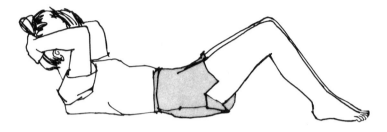

Figure 13

stretch along your neck and upper back (see Fig. 13). Hold the position for a few seconds, then lower your head to the floor. Do only three of these at first, then gradually work up to five.

**Shoulder Stand.** This is the most difficult of the exercises, but it does more for you than just untense the neck and shoulders. According to yoga teachers, it allows the blood to flow into the thyroid gland and improves its functioning. Also, it gets more blood into the brain so that you can think better, and that's a welcome advantage to headachoholics who spend so many hours hardly capable of thinking at all. However, this exercise is not recommended for women with hypertension or cardiovascular pulmonary problems. In fact, there are several physical maladies that might be exacerbated by this exercise. So it would be a good idea to check with your doctor before trying it.

Lie down on a mat or towel. Place your hands along your sides, palms down. Slowly lift your legs, knees straight and together, and when they're high enough so that it's time to bend at the hips, move your hands up under your hips to brace yourself while you swing your legs into a vertical position (see Fig. 14). When you're in the correct position, your chin will be almost touching your chest. With your elbows on the floor and hands

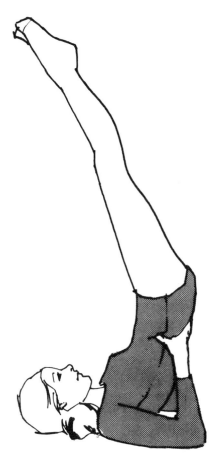

Figure 14

bracing your hips, just remain standing on your shoulders for at least twenty seconds. Those who do yoga regularly can hold this position as long as three minutes at a time.

**The Plough.** This is an extension of the shoulder stand. When you reach the point where you're standing on your shoulders, swing your legs backward with your toes pointing toward the floor. To brace yourself, put your arms on the floor with the palms of your hands down. Keeping your legs straight, lower your toes as far toward the floor

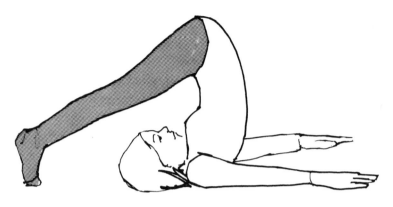

Figure 15

as you can without straining or hurting (see Fig. 15). Stay in this position for the count of ten. Feel the stretch all along your spine. Roll out of the position and lower your legs to the floor without raising your head. The more you do this exercise the closer your toes will come to the floor until they finally touch.

If these exercises make you feel as good as we think they will, you may want to do more of them and stretch your entire body. To help you do this you can order an easy-to-follow chart, "Everyday Stretches" from stretching, P.O. Box 2734, Fullerton, CA 92633 for $2.00 plus 35¢ postage.

You may also want to sign up for a yoga course at your local community college or recreation department. You can also check the program guide of the educational TV channel in your area to see if they have either Richard Hittleman's "Yoga for Health" series or "Lilias, Yoga, and You."

## AEROBIC EXERCISES

Aerobic exercises condition the heart, lungs, and blood vessels while increasing the body's ability to utilize oxygen and thereby ward off the cardiovascular diseases such as heart attack and stroke that plague the modern world.

Aerobic exercises also have special and specific benefits for chronic headache sufferers, including total cure in some cases.

There are several types of exercise that fall into the category of aerobic: bicycling, swimming, rowing, cross-country skiing, and running. But for our purposes the most significant of these is running. It can be done anywhere, anytime, by anyone, and with hardly any equipment. In short, it is the accessible aerobic. It is for this reason that running has been used in headache treatment experiments. It is also for this reason that we run ourselves and recommend it to you.

**Running**

According to Dr. Otto Appenzeller, a headache specialist in New Mexico, all headaches, except those from such causes as meningitis and tumor, can be almost totally cured by running. So no matter whether you're vascular or muscular or a combination headachoholic, he believes running can work for you and, in fact, even stomp that demon, classic migraine, to earth. In his clinic he treats headache victims with running therapy and makes them both headache-free and medication-free.

Running as a cure for headaches has been verified by others. Dr. Joan Ullyot, a San Francisco physician and now a marathon runner, used to have regular headaches that came on twice a month and lasted about two days each. Since she took up running five years ago she hasn't had a headache.

One man whose case was reported in the November 1977 issue of *Headache* discovered he usually had headaches only during quiescent periods and never when he was physically active. The next time he felt the headache warning signs of pressure starting to build in his head, he ran 220 yards in twenty-five seconds. Within three minutes the pressure was gone and no pain developed. Another time he awakened at night with a headache. He got out of bed, ran in place, and within a few minutes the pain went away. After those experiences he has always used exercise to abort his headaches and claims that "usually one running session is enough and the pain stops within five minutes."

Dr. Heuser advises his vascular headache patients who feel well enough to do so to try to "run away from their headaches." If you're going to do this you should begin running at the first hint of a headache—just about the same time you'd ordinarily take Cafergot.

Why is running able to abort or, if done consistently, totally cure headaches? Like everything else about headaches there is an element of mystery to this and a number of possible explanations. We've developed a personal theory that running may continually massage the foot reflexology and acupressure points in the feet.

Dr. Appenzeller offers some more scientific speculations. One is that activities like running increase the production of monoamine oxidase (MAO), an enzyme that keeps blood vessels in the brain from expanding. Another possibility, he says, is that the increased oxygen that endurance exercise draws into the body helps relieve headaches. Running also creates the relaxation response that, Dr. Appenzeller thinks, is not too different from that attained by yoga, hypnosis, meditation, and the like—a toning down of the autonomic nervous system.

He believes, too, that since most tension headaches are associated with depression, running helps by improving your mood. In fact, a British research team headed by Dr. Malcolm Carruthers discovered that a hormone—norepinephrine—that literally raises your spirits is released in the body by only ten minutes of intensive exercise. You might call it the happy hormone.

Another possible reason for the effectiveness of running in headache therapy is that it is truly holistic—it works on every part of you, neglecting nothing. Every dedicated runner will tell you that your whole life changes along with your body when you embark upon a rigorous running program. Bad habits like smoking, drinking, overeating, and generally carousing around seem to magically go away of their own accord. If you take up running seriously, you will undoubtedly lose weight along with your headaches and begin looking as well as feeling better. You will, in sum, become a new, improved you and this is exactly the kind of total life change that, as we've pointed out, a headache sufferer needs.

But what about the "dangers" of running? If you've read books on running, you know that most of them recommend going to the doctor for a stress test before embarking on a running program. But the famous running doctor, George Sheehan, says you only need a stress test if you're going to sit around and do nothing all the time, because that's what *really* stresses the body. At any rate, as a chronic headache sufferer you've probably had enough physical examinations to know that you don't have any kind of heart problem that would keep you from running.

**Equipment.** Now if our sales pitch has convinced you to give running away from your headaches a try, how do you start? First off, we suggest a good pair of training shoes. (If there are no specialized stores for running shoes in your area you can write to Starting Line Sports, Box 8, Mountain View, CA 94042 for their *Complete Runner's Catalog*, which contains a fine selection of shoes and directions on how to order the correct size. You can also write to Spiridon Athletic Equipment, P.O. Box 170, Allston, MA 02134 for their catalog.) When trying on shoes be sure to wear the socks that you intend to wear when you run.

Please, we beg you, don't use tennis shoes for running. They don't position your feet properly and don't protect you from the jars and jolts of the road or sidewalk or track or ground. These jars, caused by the wrong shoes, are transmitted all through your body right up to and including your vulnerable head.

Aside from the shoes, you can wear anything that's loose

and comfortable and appropriate to the weather. One clothing warning comes from Dr. Jack Skaff, head of the Honolulu Marathon Clinic. If you find your fingers are swollen after a run, it means your bra is too tight. He believes that you should run without a bra if you can do so comfortably. Otherwise he recommends a bikini top.

**Your Running Program.** Now to launch into your running program. For it to work, you should run seven to nine miles at a speed of seven to nine minutes per mile. This of course is a general guide. Dr. Appenzeller finds some headache sufferers may require twelve miles while others need only five. Although many runners believe you should have a day or two of body rest a week, Dr. Appenzeller tells his patients to run *every day*. Seven to nine miles every day at that brisk pace is your ultimate goal for the most effective headache relief. For now we're just going to sneak you into running at your body's own pace, combining walking with running.

Any running book (see Suggested Reading) can give you information on when, where, and how to run and what stretching exercises to do. What we are interested in is telling you how to start your running program with the goal of relieving your headaches. The following method is one that June finds workable and effective.

When you first begin your program, do it for only fifteen minutes. June prefers to work with time rather than distance. If you have as your goal a certain number of miles, you may try to run faster to get them over with and get back to some project that's hanging over your head. This destroys the whole conditioning and relaxing aspects of the routine.

Our basic rule and one that June always tries to follow is to walk as fast as possible and run as slowly as possible.

Walk briskly for about five minutes, then run very slowly at what's called "a conversational pace." This means you're running slowly enough to carry on a conversation without getting out of breath. When your very slow run-

ning starts to make you feel tired and winded, go back to
your very fast walking.

And that's all there is to it. Keep at it every day (or with
one or two days a week off), gradually increasing the total
time and the amount of that time you spend running
rather than walking. Your body will tell you when to make
the increases. When you find you can run the whole
fifteen minutes, add five or ten minutes of walking at the
beginning and end of your outing. Then gradually up the
running to half an hour with five or ten minutes of walking before and after. It will not be too terribly long before
you're running an hour and that will probably figure out
at an easy twelve-minute-mile pace for five miles, only two
miles and three minutes per mile short of Dr. Appenzeller's magic numbers for headache cure.

You may wonder what to do with your mind while
you're doing all this with your body. Well, what you
shouldn't do is stew over your problems and sort through
all the things you should be doing instead of "wasting
your time" running. That builds up the kind of headache-inducing stress that even a nine-mile run might
have trouble overcoming.

What June does is to combine meditation with running.
Chant your mantra, count your exhalations, or do whatever best cleanses your mind of its incessant woe-
churnings.

Before we run down we feel obliged to mention that
there are some reports of running bringing on headaches.
These are, however, usually reports from non-headache
sufferers who are intense runners and not from sedentary
sorts with a history of chronic headaches. Dr. Appenzeller
believes these headaches to be exertion headaches that are
caused by the stress of competition—even competition
against yourself—or by the dehydration that can accom-
pany slow long-distance runs.

For headache sufferers, the greatest risk is not the harm
you could do yourself by running, but the help you deny

yourself by not giving running a try as a headache cure. Even Dr. Appenzeller admits that only very few headache patients have the necessary discipline and perseverance to achieve the endurance levels necessary for a total cure. As Dr. Joan Ullyot, who knows from experience, says, "The hardest step for a women who wants to run is the first one out the door because she has to lay aside all her old ways of thinking."

Now that you've laid aside your old ways of thinking about exercise, it's time for you to pick up some new holistic ways of thinking that can reduce headache-triggering stress.

# 7

## STRESS-REDUCING TECHNIQUES FOR THE MIND

It was only after her TMJ diagnosis that June thought of practicing certain of these stress-reducing techniques. This was rather like locking the barn door after the stolen horse had been returned so that it wouldn't get stolen again. She has chosen a combination of autogenics (self-hypnosis) and meditation with occasional sessions of guided imagery. Do they work? Well, as you know, her headaches are gone, and who's to say how much credit can be given to the eight crowns Dr. Greene put in her mouth and how much to what she's doing on her own. One thing we *can* vouch for: A combination of the body techniques from Chapter 6 and the mind techniques in this chapter can give you the holistic view of yourself and of your life that will enable you to take charge of your headache.

We're going to give you instruction in four unstressing therapies: autogenics, meditation, biofeedback, and guided imagery. Only you can decide which ones seem to be right for you. There is no proven difference in their effectiveness. When we were investigating them, we came across a fascinating scientific phenomenon. In journals devoted exclusively to biofeedback, this was the treatment that did most for eliminating headaches; in journals specializing in hypnosis, autogenics (self-hypnosis) turned out to be superior to all the other therapies. And so it went. One important fact we did uncover was that the best results are obtained by combining two or more of these therapies, just as June has done.

A final tip is that you get results from these therapies only if you adopt a "let it happen" attitude. Paradoxically, the less you try, the greater your progress. How do you manage to soft sell these therapies to yourself? The directions we've read include such admonitions as, "Have a creatively expectant attitude," "Use passive volition," "Make effortless effort," "Plant the seed and let it grow." But perhaps the most graphic and understandable description we've come across is the one that compares the method of performing these techniques to urination: "Just relax and let go."

## AUTOGENIC TRAINING

Autogenics—the word means self-generating—is a tension-relieving method that involves repeating short self-hypnotic sentences to yourself in order to influence your body to relax. For example, "my right arm is very heavy" is the first suggestion you give your body to help your muscles relax. You concentrate first on creating feelings of heaviness and then of warmth. Feelings of heaviness indicate relaxed muscles and warmth means your blood vessels have dilated (relaxed). Once your right arm is heavy and warm, the body communicates this message to other muscles and you slip into a generalized total-body state of relaxation.

Autogenic training was perfected in Europe in the 1930s by a German doctor, J. H. Schultz, and has been widely known and used as a therapy there, but it is only now catching on in the U.S. In Europe the training is usually given by physicians. Americans are being introduced to it through pain clinics and self-help books.

We're going to teach you the autogenic training formulas in stages, because that's the best way to learn them, in fact, the only way to learn them. To do this we divided Dr. Schultz's original script into six parts: (1) heavy arms and legs, (2) warm arms and legs, (3) calm heartbeat, (4) regular breathing, (5) warm abdomen, and (6) cool forehead. We recorded a cassette tape of the entire autogenic relaxation script and used it ourselves over a period of several weeks, and we tried the tape on several friends. We found that it works well for almost every accepting person who does not close her mind to self-hypnosis.

In the beginning you are supposed to practice three times a day—after lunch and dinner and before bed. You can either lie down on a couch or bed with a pillow under your head and neck and assume the corpse position or you can sit in a highbacked straight chair.

Close your eyes, breathe deeply, and exhale slowly a few times to get general body relaxation, and then *slowly* repeat to yourself the following sentences. As you say each sentence, concentrate on that part of your body and imagine or feel it doing what you are telling it to do.

**Stage 1: Heaviness**
My right arm is heavy. (Repeat each sentence four times.)
My left arm is heavy.
Both arms are heavy.
My right leg is heavy.
My left leg is heavy.
**Stage 2: Warmth**
My right arm is warm. (Repeat each sentence four times.)
My left arm is warm.
Both arms are warm.

My right leg is warm.

My left leg is warm.

**Stage 3: Calm Heartbeat**

My heartbeat is calm and regular. (Repeat four times.)

**Stage 4: Regular Breathing**

My body breathes itself. (Repeat four times.)

**Stage 5: Warm Abdomen**

My abdomen is warm. (Repeat four times.)

**Stage 6: Cool Forehead**

My forehead is cool. (Repeat four times.)

At the end of each of your practice sessions, you have to bring yourself back to an active state, cancelling or deactivating the training formulas by saying, "Arms firm, breathe deeply, open eyes." You have to be very careful not to forget this cancelling sentence or you'll be trying to go about your regular activities with various parts of your body semihypnotized.

It may take you no time at all—only a session or two—to get through stages 1 and 2 and warm your arms and legs. And then again it may take you several weeks. We have to be vague, because it all depends on how suggestible you are. Some people, and Barbara is one of these, have only to let a thought walk once across their minds and the body picks it up and goes into action. Not surprisingly, it took Barbara only one session of autogenics to be able to warm her hands to the point of practically being able to fry eggs on them. June's suggestibility was initially much lower, but with practice she's increased her mind power amazingly.

Spend as much time as you need on each stage in order to master it completely before going on and adding the next one. When you can go through the entire sequence of formulas from heavy arms to cool forehead in under five minutes, you can abbreviate the sequence into, "My arms and legs are heavy and warm ... heartbeat calm and regular ... my body breathes itself ... my abdomen is warm ... my forehead is cool ..." plus the cancelling formula, "Arms firm, breathe deeply, open eyes."

When you advance to this point you can add additional autosuggestions of your own devising, such as "My forehead is cool and pain-free."

We'd like to warn you not to get discouraged if you experience the slipping-back syndrome. That is, you may seem to deteriorate in your ability to respond to these self-commands, but with continued practice you will surge ahead again. Also, there is the possibility of what are known as "autogenic discharges" during the practice sessions. These are such things as muscle twitching, trembling, crying spells, and nausea. They're perfectly normal when unstressing, and meditators experience them, too. Just don't feel frightened if they should happen to you.

As you learned in Chapter 5, hand warming is a proven technique for aborting and controlling vascular headaches. The autogenic formulas, if you're a very good student, allow you to raise your hand temperature by as much as three degrees.

What we ourselves particularly like about the training, since hand warming wasn't all that important to us when we were experimenting with this technique, was the total body relaxation we could achieve with it. In fact, we both still use autogenic formulas for putting ourselves to sleep at night after a tension-filled day or for putting ourselves back to sleep if we wake up in the early morning hours.


## MEDITATION

Meditation comes out of Eastern mystical tradition. We're concerned here not with the complex centuries-old religious teachings of Buddhism associated with meditation, but with some basic meditation exercises.

Meditation doesn't focus you on any specific body process to change it the way autogenics and biofeedback do. It is a generalized unstressing technique that releases you from your thinking machine, from that restless voice inside your head that never lets up on you except when you're asleep or unconscious. What we particularly like about meditation for women with headaches is that if you can carry it off, it gives you a wonderful respite from that problem you carry around in your thoughts all your waking hours—your headache. To put meditation in perspective, we understand that it does for your brain waves what biofeedback training does for them when you're hooked up to an alpha-wave feedback machine. We will explain biofeedback in the next section, but many of you probably know that with training you learn to generate more alpha waves (the slow ones associated with states of relaxation) and therefore to be less anxious and tense. The difference is that with biofeedback you learn to control your brain waves more quickly than you do through meditation, because the signal tells you exactly how you're progressing. (The corollary to this, of course, is that when you're unplugged from the machine you may not be able to maintain this control.)

Meditation is slower than biofeedback but the end result is the same, except that meditation possibly gives more lasting benefits, and you stand to gain much more than just control of your hand temperature and your alpha waves. If you practice consistently, meditation can change not just your physiology but your entire life.

It's our impression that some doctors shy away from recommending meditation because of its religious implications. June chose it entirely on her own. She has great faith in it and would like to pass on her own chosen description of what it is. This is from *The Mantram Handbook* by Eknath Easwaran, a Hindu teacher who founded the Blue Mountain Center of Meditation in Berkeley, California.

[Meditation] is not a religion; it is a technique which enables us to realize for ourselves the unity of life within any of the world's great religious traditions, or even if we profess no religion at all. There is a popular misconception that meditation is making your mind a blank, or wool-gathering, or letting your mind wander around some theme. Meditation is anything but these; it is a dynamic discipline in concentration which enables us to unify our consciousness completely.

## Busy Doing Nothing

The objective in all meditation is to control the attention. What you do is block out the outer world and submerge yourself in your own inner world. Each school of Buddhism, each branch of each school, even each yogi or Zen master seems to have his own set of instructions for how to do it. Transcendental Meditation (TM) is the meditative technique most of us have heard about, because it's been well publicized and advertised in the U.S. by its founder, Maharishi Mahesh Yogi. In TM you restrict your attention by repeating a sound (mantra) over and over again while sitting with your eyes closed. TM is based on an East Indian form of Buddhism. In Zen, the Japanese form of Buddhism, you open up your attention by concentrating on your breathing.

We're going to discuss here only the beginning exercises for each of these two types of meditation. And what we tell you may sound simplistic, but, believe us, only the explanation *is* simplistic. The process itself is extremely elusive and takes dedication to master. Until you've tried it, you can't realize how almost utterly impossible it is to harness your mind or turn it off for even a few seconds, let alone for half an hour. (You *can* do it, however.) Nor can you realize what a stunning relief it is from your normal state of awareness when you finally manage to do it, even briefly.

**Mantra Meditation.** Let's begin with transcendental—mantra or sound—meditation and then go on to Zen—breathing—meditation. The first step is to choose your sound. The mantra is usually short, as short as a single syllable or two. It should have a melodious sound. The TMers say it should have no special significance, but in much Hindu yoga practice the mantra is often an inspirational passage of several syllables or even words. Patricia Carrington, a Princeton University psychologist who uses meditation for mental therapy in her counseling practice, suggests that students in her program pick whichever of the following mantras sounds to them most pleasant and soothing: Ah-nam, Shi-rim, or Ra-mah. Or, if you insist on spending $165, you can sign up for a Maharishi Mahesh Yogi TM course and you will be assigned the particular mantra that is "perfect" for you and must be kept secret. (Patricia Carrington says the TM mantras are not all that special; in fact, she has found out they are assigned according to your age.)

To do your mantra meditation, you go to your chosen spot and take your chosen position. Take a few slow, deep breaths to quiet yourself, but not so deep that you become lightheaded. Then close your eyes and start repeating your mantra slowly to yourself over and over again, breathing through your nose and breathing abdominally. As extraneous thoughts and images crowd into your mind, let them flow through without allowing them to distract you from concentrating on your mantra. It's something like placing yourself in an isolation chamber. As with the other unstressing techniques, it's virtually an impossibility to explain how to do it. In fact, some Indian teachers say that you don't "do" it. You create in yourself a state of nondoing and meditation happens spontaneously.

When you finish, you stop repeating the mantra and sit several minutes with your eyes still closed. Rather than snapping yourself out of your meditative state, you open your eyes, stretch the way you would when awaking from a nap, and then get up and resume your normal activities. You will feel refreshed, energized, never tense, and, we hope, headache-free.

**Zen Meditation.** Turning now to Zen technique, how you sit is very important. Use the full or half lotus or sit on the forward part of a straight chair. Your spine should be straight and the small of your back concave (abdomen pushed out), your chin pulled in. Hands in your lap and turned up with left inside right, unless you're lefthanded; in that case, right inside left. Thumbs lightly touching. Eyes open looking about three feet in front of you and downward but unfocused. Begin by moving your torso in a wide circle, gradually narrowing the circle until you come to stop at your natural center, where you will feel balanced and secure.

Now you must sit there and let your mind follow the movement of your breathing. You must use abdominal breathing. In and out, in and out. You let other thoughts and images come but you also let them go, as you continue concentrating on your breathing. You can count one as you exhale if this helps, or one as you inhale and two as you exhale. You can even count your breathing clear up to ten, but no higher, as this is distracting. Eventually you get to the point that you can just sit and feel your breathing without counting. In fact, Zen teachers (*roshis*) refer to Zen practice as "just sitting."

**Where and When to Meditate.** Meditation should always be practiced in the same place, someplace where you will not be interrupted and where there is no noise. Finding this serene atmosphere is often the biggest challenge. June uses a small dining room that looks out onto the patio.

There are numerous traditional positions for meditation. Figures 16, 17, and 18 demonstrate three good possibilities. Select the one most comfortable for you personally.

June finds it a good practice to meditate at the same time each day. She then looks forward to this time as free from stress. Early morning on arising and before breakfast is the best time for her and for most women. (Meditating after eating is not recommended.) Before dinner is good, also, but before bed is not (it may heighten your consciousness to the point that you cannot get to sleep).

Start with five minutes a day and gradually extend the time until you can handle as much as one-half hour. June has been meditating off and on for ten months and she has never gone over fifteen minutes. A short meditation done daily is far preferable to a longer one done erratically. And if you have to change time or place occasionally, do so rather than eliminating that day's practice entirely.

Many meditators feel that for any form of meditation you should work under the direction of a teacher, because you need someone to answer your questions and help you with uncomfortable emotional and physical side effects that appear as you are becoming unstressed, the same as with autogenics. Our suggestion for finding a teacher is to check with community and four-year colleges in your vicinity. Many offer courses in meditation with the classes sometimes meeting at the headquarters of yoga or Zen training centers. We have also noticed that meditation with a Christian emphasis is offered in some churches. You can find announcements about these sessions in your local newspaper.

## BIOFEEDBACK

Biofeedback is a new science only eight or ten years old. In biofeedback training, electronic instruments are used to feed back to you information about what is happening inside your body. Using this information, you learn to modify your own internal body processes such as your blood pressure, pulse rate, temperature, and muscle tension.

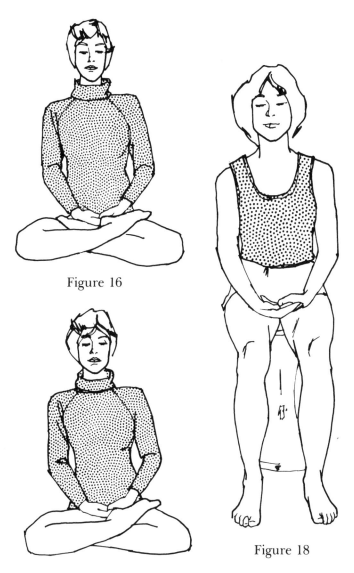

Figure 16

Figure 17

Figure 18

Biofeedback has emerged strongly onto the headache-control scene during the last few years. Dr. Janos Kalla of the Department of Anesthesiology, School of Medicine, UCLA, stated in a lecture that biofeedback is only 40 percent effective for headaches, unless it is combined with either autogenics or deep-muscle-relaxation exercises. In this case the rate rises to 80 percent. But no matter what biofeedback can or cannot do for the pain of headache, it's convincing doctors that holistic therapies do work. They are accepting it as a legitimate treatment, and more and more of them are purchasing the instruments needed to provide biofeedback treatment in their own offices. Dr. Heuser had recommended it to June if she was not going to have her bite adjusted by Dr. Greene.

In the biofeedback teaching sessions there is always a trainer who guides you through the process of learning how to control your muscle tension, temperature, brain waves, pulse rate, etc. The training requires that you visit a doctor's office or biofeedback laboratory for an uninterrupted period of seven to twelve weeks. The sessions usually last at least thirty minutes each and are scheduled for once a day or once or twice a week. Also, you are required to practice the skills you acquire regularly at home or no learning is possible.

There are several different kinds of feedback information used and several different kinds of machines. Your trainer decides which one or ones are best for you. These are the possibilities:

**EMG—Electromyogram.** The electromyogram measures muscle tension. Electrodes are placed in the center of the forehead about an inch above the eyebrows. This allows the instrument, the electromyograph, to check tension in the frontalis muscle, a forehead muscle thought to be the best indicator of tension in the head and neck and shoulders. The EMG can be used for all kinds of headaches, since no matter what the cause, all headaches create at least reflex muscle tension in the head and adjacent muscles.

**EEG—Electroencephalogram.** This shows brain wave patterns as measured by an electroencephalograph. EEG biofeedback is used to train you to produce alpha and theta brain waves. These are the slower brain rhythms associated with mental states of tranquility (nonheadache states). With EEG, electrodes are placed on the head.

**GSR—Galvanic Skin Response.** This is another gauge of how relaxed a person is. The galvanometer measures the skin's resistance to electricity. Your skin's resistance to electricity goes down when you perspire and it becomes wet. Therefore, the more tenseness, the less resistance and the more prone you are to headaches. (This instrument is also used as a lie detector.) You are hooked up to it by electrodes placed on the hands.

**Temperature.** Thermometers are used on the hands to let you know whether you are raising or lowering their temperature. A special temperature training device can be used or a simple thermometer, the bulb of which is taped to your finger.

In biofeedback training sessions your hands and/or your head are hooked up to one or more of these instruments, which tell you by means of a light that goes on and off or gets brighter or dimmer what is happening in your body. Sometimes a sound that gets softer or louder is used as a signal.

Emile White, a colleague of ours at Los Angeles Valley College, was an early biofeedback trainee for headache control. She had had headaches virtually every day since she started menstruating at the age of thirteen. For years she had used Cafergot with PB (suppository type) to control her headaches. In 1976 she saw a brochure from her health service (Ross-Loos) about biofeedback. She asked her doctor to refer her to the program, as she was anxious to reduce her dependence on drugs.

First, she was required to take a written psychological examination to see if she was a good candidate for training. (Not everyone is. You have to believe you can integrate your mind and body.) They accepted her and she stayed with it for the full ten-week training period. She went once a week for one hour. They attached her to three instruments—EEG, EMG, and a hand thermometer. Of these, she was told hand temperature was the most important for her. As she raised the temperature of her hands, a sound signal would get lower and lower. Absolute quiet meant she was doing nicely. She learned to raise the temperature of her hands in one minute and could abort her headache about 75 percent of the time by the end of the ten weeks.

During the learning period she had three different trainers. To her mind, it was the skill of the trainer that made the big difference. Only with her third trainer did she make progress, because he used abdominal breathing exercises—normal intakes combined with very slow exhales—to get her relaxed enough to learn. Only after these breathing exercises plus some progressive relaxation exercises did he attach the machines. He stayed in the room with her the entire time and would give her assurances such as "Whatever it is you're doing now, keep doing it."

We asked Emile to explain to us exactly what were her mental directions to her body in order to change the temperature of her hands. At first, she put herself in a serene state by looking at some posters that were on the office wall—a sea view and a picture of a person on a hill overlooking a valley. These scenes helped her create mental images of places of relaxation.

Then she switched to thinking about warming her hands. She imagined putting them on an old-fashioned potbellied stove or holding them in front of an open fire.

Later she progressed to the stage that she just thought of warm hands and got results. She imagined warm, tingling sensations in her fingertips. She found thinking of hot fingertips worked better than concentrating on her entire hand.

After Emile could warm her hands without using the thermometer—she had weaned herself away from the feedback information—she was considered a successful student and no longer had to report for training. She was given another written test that showed she had definitely reduced her anxiety. She had, in fact, also reduced her headaches.

Following the ten-week course Emile used hand temperature control at home every day for a while. But her problem was fear. Her headaches came on between 3:00 A.M. and 5:00 A.M. in the morning. If she tried biofeedback and failed then she was in for a two- or three-day seige. If she took her Cafergot, she knew she could escape the headache. So if she really needed to function well she felt she could not take the risk of biofeedback. Then, to keep in training she had to practice raising her hand temperature every day, and she simply couldn't get enough time to practice.

In spite of these obstacles, Emile considered her training a success, because it allowed her to cut the amount of medication she was using by one half and gave her headache relief much of the time. And she still uses hand warming whenever she feels it can help her.

As we see it, for those of you who are hesitant about trying your ability to integrate mind and body and control your headaches from within, biofeedback training is a perfect bridge. It's the scientific approach to the unscientific. But it has several drawbacks:

1. You have to locate a reliable service.
2. You must be willing to commit yourself to weeks of appointments.
3. The training is expensive and is not (at this writing) covered by medical insurance, al-

though some health insurance groups, such as Ross-Loos, do offer it to subscribers.

4. You can get hooked on the machines—figuratively—and find it hard to make the transition from them to yourself.

As for availability of biofeedback, here in our area of Southern California we are bombarded with advertisements for biofeedback training by independent laboratories. These charge about $50 a session and require that you sign up for a minimum of ten sessions in the beginning. Some headache specialists and clinics offer biofeedback in their own offices for much less than independent laboratories.

If your doctor cannot advise you about biofeedback training services, contact the Biofeedback Society of America, Department of Psychiatry C268, University of Colorado Medical Center, 4200 East Ninth Avenue, Denver, CO 80220 and ask for their list of certified members.

## GUIDED IMAGERY

Guided imagery or visualization, as some pain therapists call it, is forming images in your mind to achieve a healing effect. This technique offers you two important benefits. First, it allows you to escape from your daily tensions into a tranquil haven, and second, once there, through the eyes of an advisor you are at last able to look at the big picture of the whole integrated mind-body-environment complex of your life and see what out-of-focus elements are responsible for your headaches.

As a holistic technique of self-therapy, guided imagery has very respected credentials among pain therapists and psychologists. And recent studies of the brain's hemispheres are helping scientists understand how guided imagery works.

The brain has two hemispheres. The left hemisphere

controls the right side of the body; the right hemisphere controls the left. The left hemisphere is the verbal, logical half. The right hemisphere is where your intuition and creativity abide. This side works not with words, but with pictures, with images. Some scientists believe that the right half also controls the body's perception of pain. Consequently, it just could be that when it comes to pain control, one guided imagery picture from the right hemisphere is worth a thousand words from the left.

One pain therapist has noticed a strange hemispheric phenomenon. Patients who have pain exclusively on the right side of the body are the hardest ones to work with and cure. It could be that they are almost totally dominated by their left hemisphere. Guided imagery is designed to awaken the right hemisphere. It is a perfect path to holistic consciousness.

## Girl Guide

As the name of the technique suggests, you need a guide to lead you along this path. We're going to introduce you to such a guide, to someone who can really help you, to a wise woman advisor. No, it's not either of us. She's a person who knows much more about you than we ever could. Here's how you go about meeting her.

Think about a calm and beautiful place, a place where you have been contented and at ease. It could be in the mountains or beside the sea or a lake or a stream or in the desert or the woods, anywhere that you feel in harmony with yourself and the world.

Close your eyes and go there. Visualize yourself walking into this calming place. Hear the sounds, smell the aromas, touch the foliage or the sand or the grass, feel the warmth or the cool. Experience it with body and mind. Sit down and rest for a while, enveloped by the peace.

Gradually become aware that you are not alone. There is someone sitting nearby. It is a woman. She is wise and kind. She is all-knowing, all-understanding, all-forgiving.

Perhaps she's someone out of your past—your grandmother, an aunt, a teacher or counselor. Or perhaps she's someone you've never met and yet you know her and she knows you. You know you can rely on her to help you.

You smile at her. She smiles back. You talk for a while. You ask her if she will help you find some answers. She says of course she will.

You ask her a question. Perhaps it's not the most important question of your life at this early stage of your relationship, but still it's an important question, something you need to know in order to heal yourself. Wait for her answer. Give her time to think and respond. She will respond.

Continue to sit calmly and think about what she has told you with all of its possible meanings.

When you feel you have truly understood her message, thank her and embrace her warmly before you depart. Tell her you look forward to returning and talking with her again soon.

As you leave your peaceful place, you feel joyful, fulfilled, healthy, loving, and that most nebulous and sought-after of conditions, happy.

Visit your peaceful place and your wise woman until she answers all your life questions. She will tell you what changes you need to make and she will give you the courage and strength to make them.

The advisor in guided imagery can be a woman or a man or a child or even an animal. June actually had a golden seal named Benigna, who sat with her in the mental coves of an imaginary Laguna Beach and gave her life counsel.

Perhaps you have already figured out who this advisor really is: she is your own inner wisdom. After all, only you have the knowledge and insight to answer the important questions you're going to be asking about yourself and your life. With guided imagery you can open a wonderful new communication between your conscious and unconscious minds and solve many problems, including your headache problems, through your own creativity.

## SOME TIME FOR YOURSELF
With all of these unstressing techniques the most important and the hardest part is taking the time to do them. Sometimes it doesn't matter so much which method you choose as it does that you get out from under your routines and pressures and demands while you're practicing whatever it is you prefer.

Some quiet moments alone just doing five minutes of deep abdominal breathing (inhale for a count of three, hold for three, exhale for a count of three) can help. So can good old-fashioned daydreaming. Let your mind roll onto whatever pleasant spot you like and picture yourself doing whatever pleasant activity you most enjoy.

Women have particular difficulty carving out time for themselves. If they're mothers, it can be almost impossible. As one mother of four told us, "Children are very selfish. You have to accept that. Mother is just there to be used." She herself hides in the bathroom to meditate, and she's trained her children that she's not to be interrupted for *anything* for her sacred twenty minutes.

You must have heard by now the basic psychological truth that before you can love others, you have to love yourself. There are other related truths for you as a headache sufferer to remember: You have to take in order to be able to give. You have to be selfish in order to be selfless. You have to help yourself in order to be the most help to others.

Help yourself out of your pain.

# 8

## HOLISTIC HEADACHE SPECIALISTS AND PAIN CLINICS

For many headache sufferers the most efficient way to help themselves out of their pain—in fact, sometimes the *only* way—is to do what June did: to put themselves in the care of a *holistic headache specialist.*

Throughout this book we have been helping you help yourself by gathering clues, keeping a headache diary, and practicing both immediate and far-reaching relief and destressing techniques. You may have already cured your headaches by yourself. But if you haven't, you now have the information that a holistic doctor needs if you are both to collaborate on your cure.

Going to a headache specialist is, in a sense, like hiring a Sherlock Holmes or a James Bond to help you with your investigation. It's much easier than digging out all the clues, following up on all the leads by yourself. Also, you must admit that physicians have access to information you don't have and have the experience you lack. And a holistic doctor will pool resources with you as you both search for a cure.

We can almost hear your groans of protest: "But I've been to ____ number of doctors already." (One woman we read about filled in that ____ with the number 97!) "I've tried every one of their therapies, every one of their drugs, but I have just as much pain as ever and a lot less money."

You probably also have a lot less faith in doctors than you did in the beginning, even as June does. Over her years of medical adventures from tonsillectomy to hysterectomy to diabetes to headaches, she gradually lost most of her former reverence for health professionals.

During the disillusioned periods of her headache-cure odyssey June kept muttering that the Chinese have the only logical approach to the medical establishment. They pay their doctors not for treating them when they're ill but for keeping them well. And in the last months of her ordeal she came to prefer the Shoshone system. After three patients die, they bump off the medicine man.

Now having come full circle and owing her cure to men with medical and dental degrees, June's perspective is slightly different. Her new view is best expressed as a Zen riddle. She has total faith in doctors, yet she has no faith in them. Doctors can be wondrous allies in your struggle for health—or they can be saboteurs who undermine your efforts. It all depends on the skill and dedication of the individual doctor and on your ability to interact holistically with him.

So no matter how few or how many doctors you've already seen, no matter how much or how little faith you now have in the profession, we still think there is another doctor in your future—the one who can diagnose the cause or causes of your headaches and help you rid yourself of them, the one you've got to find.

If you still feel you've already tried every kind of treatment and have been defeated, ask yourself this: Did you give up before the new headache-as-a-disease approach came onto the scene, before headache treatment became an area of specialization for doctors? In other words, have you really exhausted all the *present* medical possibilities?

## DOC WORK: THE HOLISTIC HEADACHE SPECIALIST

Even if you decide to hire a fellow detective—your doctor—you can't escape detective work entirely because it takes a fair amount of investigation just to find the headache specialist you/need. Headache specialists are certainly not practicing on every street corner or in every town or even in every major city, but they *can* be found if you put your mind to it.

First, let's clear up a possible point of confusion. Sometimes doctors list themselves as headache specialists and sometimes as headache clinics or groups. (Some doctors don't like to use the term "clinic" because it sounds as if the treatment there is free.) Often the terms are interchangeable. There may be only one doctor and yet he may call his office a clinic. There may be two doctors working together who call their practice a headache clinic or a medical group. These one- and two-doctor offices probably refer their patients who require specialized treatment to physicians or therapists in other fields such as otolaryngology, dentistry, hypnosis, exercise, acupuncture, etc. Then, again, sometimes a clinic or a medical group has several kinds of specialists and therapists in association to give you all or almost all of the kinds of treatment you need on the premises.

Don't worry about the name. Be it headache specialist or headache clinic or headache medical group, it can treat you equally effectively—or poorly—depending on the skills and attitudes of the physicians and therapists involved. Usually there is one doctor in charge who sets the attitude and skill level for his staff. An outstanding director will select and keep only the best of associates. One good doctor leads to another.

Now that you can accept either a headache specialist or clinic or medical group, how then do you go about finding one in your vicinity? The first step in trying to locate one is to write the National Migraine Foundation (5214 N. Western Avenue, Chicago, IL 60625) for a list of those practicing in your area. When you receive the list, you'll also be invited to join the National Migraine Foundation. It's not a bad idea. Not only do they use the money for headache research, but they publish a newsletter that you as a member receive. It has a lot of information, both theoretical and practical, which might help you in your quest for a cure.

If the list from the Migraine Foundation doesn't include a doctor in your area, the second step is to call the local medical association and ask them if they know of a doctor who specializes in the treatment of headaches. If you strike out on that, call a nearby medical school with a teaching hospital and ask if they have a headache expert on their staff. Even if there is no one on their staff, they may be able to refer you to someone in the area whom they use for consultations.

Should there be no medical school close at hand, then get in touch with the hospital in your area that has the best reputation and ask who on their staff specializes in treating headaches. If you strike out on all these counts, follow this same routine in the nearest large city.

## A CLINICAL APPROACH: PAIN CLINICS

If you aren't able to find a headache specialist in your area, your next choice for headache detection help is a pain clinic or pain center. (In medical circles pain clinics are usually for outpatients and centers for inpatients.)

Pain clinics are staffed with a team of specialists in different fields—neurologists, orthopedists, oral surgeons, anesthesiologists, psychiatrists, social workers, etc.—and they use a wide range of therapies, including nerve blocks (blocking of nerve impulses by chemical, mechanical, or electrical means), acupuncture, biofeedback, hypnotherapy, physical therapy, group psychotherapy, psychological counseling, and various relaxation techniques.

Clinics start you off with a thorough attempt at diagnosis and a complete history. Usually in the beginning they break your pain circuit with some temporary measure, maybe even drugs, although they try to get you off them eventually.

Many use a special approach to help you change your attitude toward your pain and ease you back into normal life activities. The approach is called *operant conditioning* (behavior modification) and the way it works is that you are praised only when you ignore your pain and behave as if you didn't have it. At some clinics, like the Pain Rehabilitation Center in La Crosse, Wisconsin, you aren't even allowed to talk about your pain. Other centers try to deprogram your feelings of anxiety and self-pity by instructing you to use the word "discomfort" to refer to your pain. (As the holistic practitioners say, "What you think is how you feel.") People released from a pain clinic may still have some pain, but they will have changed their reaction to it. They will perceive it differently enough so that it will no longer disrupt their work and their lives.

Most pain clinics have a good track record for helping people overcome pain. Dr. C. Norman Shealy considers his program at the La Crosse Pain Rehabilitation Center to be successful with 80 percent of the patients. The Intractable Pain Unit at the City of Hope in Duarte, California, is one of the older and more strict programs. (The blue book for patients puts it on the line: "The changing of your pain experience will be, primarily, your responsibility.") Although 10 to 15 percent of their patients drop out, of those who finish the six-to-eight-week program, 90 percent are able to reduce their pain.

One advantage of pain clinics is that since the concept started back in the early sixties, there are more of them

than there are headache clinics. And they are prolifer-
ating at a much faster rate.

But before you decide to go off in search of a pain clinic,
there are a few things you should take into consideration.

First, unlike headache clinics, which are right on target,
pain centers treat every kind of chronic pain: low back
pain (the most common), arthritis and cancer pain,
phantom-limb pain, tic douloureux, and only *sometimes*
headache pain.

Second, pain clinics aren't always easy to get into. Since
they don't have room for every sufferer who needs help,
they have to sort out patients and accept only those who
are good candidates for the program. The Intractable
Pain Unit, for instance, will not accept a patient who is in
litigation, is considered a suicide risk, or is psychotic.
Often patients are taken only on referral from other doctors and often these are the patients their doctors consider
hopeless.

Then, too, headache sufferers sometimes are excluded
from pain clinics because there are simply too many of
them and, to quote a *Family Health* magazine article, they
are "a world of pain in themselves."

Finally, not all pain centers favor holistic medicine. In
fact, they span the entire treatment spectrum. Therefore,
you must apply the same rules in selecting a pain clinic as
you do in selecting a headache specialist. And yet, on the
other hand, you must be wary because the holistic movement has become somewhat of a lucrative bandwagon and
some unqualified practitioners are jumping onto it strictly
for commercial reasons. So if the word "holistic" is tacked
on to the name of a pain or health center, you have to be
particularly careful to investigate its scientific background
and credentials.

In Appendix D, we've included the most up-to-date and
complete guide to pain clinics that treat headache patients
that we could compile. It's still not a long list, but it's a start.
Since most pain centers are part of a university medical

school, once again we advise you to get in touch with your nearest medical school or hospital if you cannot find a nearby center on the list.

## HOLISTIC OR NOT?

Even after you locate a headache specialist, headache clinic, or pain clinic you're not quite finished with your research. As in every area of medicine, there are headache specialists and headache specialists, pain clinics and pain clinics. What you need to find is a very special specialist or clinic indeed—one with a holistic approach.

Now the idea of a holistic doctor may sound like a contradiction in terms—something rather like a pacifist general—but it's not necessarily so. Although Dr. Heuser dislikes and distrusts the commercialism of the holistic movement, he firmly believes that every *good* doctor has always practiced holism. And there are growing numbers of doctors who practice what is becoming known as integral medicine. This means they combine the modern technological and pharmacological advances of the West with the ancient wisdoms of the East; they practice both curative and preventive medicine; they mend broken bones and broken spirits. Both approaches are absolutely necessary.

As Dr. Bresler, an advocate of integral medicine, says, "If I'm run over by a truck, don't stick acupuncture needles in me. Take me to an emergency ward." He believes that there's nothing like modern Western medicine to handle the acute situation, but in the treatment of chronic pain, an area in which Western medicine has a very poor track record, Dr. Bresler uses unconventional, holistic treatments. Dr. Martin D. Shickman, director of continuing education in the health sciences at UCLA, sums it up: "Clinical medicine does not handle problems of misery very well." And as any chronic headache sufferer knows, persistent headaches are the *essence* of misery.

Holism is no longer regarded as a kooky and quacky

fad, even by the conservative American Medical Association. Whereas only a few years back an AMA president said that holism "gets into superstition, tribalism, mysticism, what we came out of 300 years ago," a recent president not only appeared at the First National Congress on Integrative Health (on the same program with an American Indian medicine man, a biofeedback expert, an acupuncturist, a psychic healer, and many other unconventionals) but also stated, "There is something here that we shouldn't turn our backs to. ... There is perhaps within the concept [of holism] an exciting rejuvenation of our health system."

If you locate a headache specialist or headache or pain clinic and want to have some idea whether it's holistically oriented or not, there is a rather obvious screening method for you to apply. You just ask. Right out loud. To see how well this direct method would work, we called the offices of two headache specialists in our area—one doctor we knew not to be holistic in his approach and one who definitely was.

We asked the receptionist in the nonholistic office if that particular clinic was holistically oriented, following up our question with a fumbling, "You know, do you use a lot of drugs and stuff like that or do you try some of the more unconventional things like acupuncture and hypnosis?"

The receptionist said, "I don't think we're what you're looking for. We use drugs and we're pretty conventional in our approach. We do use biofeedback, though."

"Oh, then biofeedback is the *only* unconventional treatment you use?"

"Yes, but we don't consider biofeedback unconventional." Then she reiterated, "I don't really think we're what you're looking for."

We considered that an honest and straightforward response.

The call to the holistic clinic worked out equally well. In reply to our query the receptionist explained that they were searching for *causes* of headaches and that they really didn't like using drugs any more than they absolutely had to. They approached the problem from all angles, using acupuncture, acupressure, biofeedback, exercise, or whatever holistic methods were appropriate for the individual case.

Using these two conversations as your guide, it would be easy to choose between the two clinics.

But stay, you are not finished with your analysis. What you have so far are words. All you can really count on are deeds. Just as the proof of the pudding is in the eating, the proof of the holistic headache specialist is in the treating.

## MDetection: A Checklist

Whether your search brings you to an individual headache specialist or a doctor practicing in a headache clinic or pain clinic, you want him to be both holistically oriented *and* a good doctor. (The two don't always go together.) In order to help you recognize whether the treatment you're getting is both holistic and good, we offer you this subjective analysis based on our experience with holistic and nonholistic doctors, with good doctors and the other kind. Since Dr. Heuser is to our admittedly biased minds the very model of a good and holistic doctor, we will frequently use him as our archetype.

*1. Does your doctor seem genuinely interested in your case and the solving of it?* We once saw Dr. Heuser, eyes shining with excitement, describe to a group of his colleagues at a headache seminar the "fun and reward" of helping a patient.

At that same seminar, Dr. Arnold Friedman, former professor of neurology at Columbia University and coauthor of *The Headache Book*, said, "The ear is more important than the eye in the diagnosis of headaches. Listen carefully. You have to have time. You have to have patience. You have to have more than a routine interest."

The time factor is especially important. Does the doctor

always keep you sitting in a crowded waiting room for one or two hours and then give you a five- or ten-minute short shift in the examining room? If so, he could be "overbooking," as they say in airline circles, to make sure he's selling his time at the maximum price. This could mean that he's more fascinated by greenbacks than by headaches.

Since we both detest waiting in doctors' offices, we'd like to be able to say that if a doctor makes you wait an hour, he's all bad and you should shun him. Unfortunately we can't. A long wait doesn't always indicate an overbooker. It may indicate a humanitarian who stops the scheduled action to help when an emergency occurs.

June had quite a long wait one time when a bathrobed woman was brought into Dr. Heuser's office with glazed eyes and a look of pain as intense as if she'd been wearing a crown of thorns. Dr. Heuser held up his other appointments to give the woman a shot of Demerol to release her from her misery. You don't — or shouldn't — mind waiting when it's one of these there-but-for-the-grace-of-God-go-I situations.

Even without emergencies, though, June sometimes had a wait of as much as an hour for Dr. Heuser. Once inside the examining room, however, he gave her his rapt attention with no eye on the clock. It figures that you may have to pay with some waiting room time for this quality and quantity of time in the examining room, since everybody is probably getting this same kind of unrushed treatment.

*2. Does the doctor regard you as an equal, or does he have a condescending attitude, conveying the idea that you are incapable of understanding your condition and its treatment?* To paraphrase novelist Kurt Vonnegut, any doctor who can't explain to an eight-year-old what he's doing is a charlatan.

A holistic doctor loves to explain and he does it in nonmedical jargon that can be easily understood. He regards himself as much teacher as healer, since in holistic medicine *you* are intended to be the one who assumes control of *your* health. A holistic doctor therefore becomes an educator who transfers knowledge and know-how to you. Biofeedback authority Barbara Brown warns that this is the hardest shift for many doctors to make, because it's a new role for them.

It's also hard for many doctors to admit their own doubts and confusions. Beware of a doctor who tries to give the impression that he's all-knowing and absolutely certain about everything he's doing. From the very beginning Dr. Heuser always admitted that he was going to try many approaches with June and that he didn't know which might succeed.

An aura of unassailable expertise in a doctor augurs a mind closed to new possibilities. What you're seeking is a knowledgeable headache expert who still thinks like a beginner, with all of the beginner's freedom and openness. In this respect it pays to remember the great Zen principle stated by Shunryu Suzuki, "In the beginner's mind there are many possibilities; in the expert's mind there are few."

A holistic doctor welcomes new possibilities, even ideas and suggestions from the patient. He is able to accept these without feeling that his authority and image are being threatened. For example, when in our research we discovered an expanded version of the low-tyramine diet, Dr. Heuser was delighted to learn about it and immediately used it to replace the less complete list he had been giving his patients.

3. *On the subject of being open to possibilities, will he try unorthodox approaches to diagnosis and treatment such as mood rings, bubblegum, megavitamins, and exercise?* The reason we feel that unorthodox approaches are necessary is that many long term headache sufferers have been exposed to every orthodox treatment in the medical textbook and these measures have generally failed.

The easiest and as a result the most commonly used

orthodox treatment for headaches is drug therapy. It is quite possible therefore that you may find yourself in the office of what we think of as a drug pusher. We once heard a psychologist explain how most physicians are taught to deal with pain: "If something hurts a little, you give an aspirin; if it hurts a little more, you give aspirin with codeine; still a little more, you give Demerol."

Now we don't mean that a good and holistic doctor never uses drugs. We mean that he uses them in conjunction with other therapies. A pusher to us is a doctor who prescribes one drug after another—tranquilizers, mood enhancers, analgesics, antihistamines—and sometimes several simultaneously ad infinitum and ad nauseam. A pusher relies totally on the pharmacopoeia to cope with your headaches and we wouldn't, if we were you, rely on him. Drugs, after all, treat only symptoms of the headache problem and, as headache expert Dr. Seymour Diamond says, "If you're being treated symptomatically, you're not being treated properly."

Another popular orthodox treatment is surgery. Be wary any time a doctor wants to cut and slice before trying other therapies to alleviate your pain. Surgery, except in those rare brain tumor cases, is notoriously ineffective for headaches. We have heard of patients who've had every nerve around the neck cut and got their headaches back again in full force after only six months of relief.

Dr. C. Norman Shealy, himself a neurosurgeon and director of the Pain Rehabilitation Center in La Crosse, Wisconsin, believes you shouldn't submit to surgery for sinus conditions, TMJ, etc., until you're certain the doctor has answered the following questions to your satisfaction:

Why is this operation "necessary"?
What are the risks of death and complications?
What are the risks *without* surgery? Are there alternative courses of treatment that don't involve surgery? What are the chances on those?

What are the chances of surgery doing what it is
supposed to do?

There's another reason for you to avoid conventional
surgery: It may reduce your chances for success with the
unconventional and less deleterious therapies. In a study
done at the UCLA Pain Control Unit, it turned out that 80
percent of the patients who had *not* undergone surgery for
pain relief gained significant relief with more unorthodox
treatments. On the other hand, only 40 percent of the
people who *had* undergone surgery before coming to the
clinic gained significant relief from their pain.

Finally, bear in mind that headache surgery is usually
elective rather than emergency. It does not involve life-
threatening conditions. In other words, you can live without it.

4. *Does the doctor seem to be mainly preoccupied with classifying
your headache and pinning a label on it?* Some doctors seem to
confuse giving a condition a name with understanding
and doing something about it. We really feel that, for
example, calling you a migraine sufferer and getting you
hooked on ergotamines (drugs like Cafergot that constrict
the blood vessels) isn't quite getting to the heart (or head)
of the matter. Actually, if all you want is a label and a drug
you needn't go to a headache specialist. *Any* doctor can
give you those.

As we mentioned, Dr. Heuser never tried to classify or
put some kind of label on June's headaches. He searched
for causes first, not categories. His motto is, "Classifying
headaches is a trap. You should only classify in retrospect."
He believes in giving the headaches a name *after* you've
cured or controlled them.

5. *Does the doctor follow the basic principle of holism in that he
takes the whole you into consideration?* Instead of the *Reader's
Digest* dissection of the body into "I am Joe's Intestine" or "I
am Jane's Womb," does he keep your body parts assem-
bled into the total person that you are? On top of that, does

he seem to realize that you have a body plus a mind plus emotions plus an environment plus a lifestyle? Does he take the entire complex of you, which is as unique as your fingerprints, and view it, not just through a microscope, but also through a telescope focused on your whole universe?

Does he then take this unique complex of you and give it a unique treatment or does he have a single form of treatment for everyone? We've heard of one clinic where almost everyone ends up on the identical drug program. This is somewhat like those beauty operators who have one hair style in their repertoire and no matter what the shape of your face or the texture of your hair, you come away from an appointment with them with exactly the same hairdo as their previous customer.

One recent book on migraine, *Control of Migraine* by Dr. John C. Brainard, claims that most migraine attacks are triggered by what you eat, and at the top of his list of taboo foods is "a sudden load of salt." The doctor himself is a migraine sufferer who noticed this salt-eating-migraine-attack connection in his own case. So his entire book is based on this factor. Sure, try a salt-free diet. It might work for you. But for *everybody*? Not likely.

Of course, after you check out all the questions on this list, you must ask the ultimate question: Does the doctor help you cure your headaches? You won't know the answer until you've tried. But of course, if he does, all other considerations go out the window. He *is* a good doctor.

## Patient, Heal Thyself

We have given you some stringent requirements to make your doctor or pain clinic meet. But holism is a two-way street. There are some equally stringent requirements for you to meet. Just as you checked out your doctor on the previous checklist, try yourself out on this one.

*1. Do you have the typical chronic pain sufferer's hostile, suspicious, negative attitude toward doctors?* Your answer to this may well be, "I sure do and with reason!" That would probably have been June's response, too—only couched in more blunt and profane terms. If you have this attitude, you're going to have to suspend it as June finally did with the doctor who cured her. If you persist in biting the hand that's trying to soothe your brow, it's almost a certainty that an alleviation or cure will be impossible.

One of our headache-suffering friends went to a specialist and was so suspicious of him that for even his most innocuous treatments, such as following a certain diet to check for food allergies, she'd run to another doctor for a second opinion. And when she talked about him she sent forth waves of hostility, waves that the doctor himself undoubtedly experienced even more intensely when he saw her in his office. Needless to say, she still has her headaches.

Negativism can be almost as bad as hostility. One pain therapist confessed to us that she felt helpless in dealing with many of her headache patients. "They get you down with their negative attitudes," she said. "Spending an hour with one of them is like spending an hour with Dracula—you feel sucked dry. How can you help people who can only see the dark side and who shoot down every possibility you offer them?" How, indeed.

*2. Will you follow your doctor's directions, do the experiments he assigns to you, follow the diet he gives you, perform the exercises he suggests?* In other words, will you cooperate with him *fully*—no slacking off and no cheating?

One patient we heard of flew all the way from Germany to see a prominent American headache specialist. After examining her the doctor told her he thought her headaches might be food-related and explained he was going to put her on a restricted diet to see if that helped.

The patient took one look at the diet, said, "I like the way I eat and I'm not going to change," got on a plane, and flew home with her headache.

Another woman, who suffered such intense headache pain that she had twice attempted suicide to escape from it, *still* refused to give up smoking even on an experimental basis.

Other patients take the sneaky way out. They pretend to be doing exactly what their doctor asks, but in reality they're cheating a lot. From our work with diabetics we're very familiar with cheating on your doctor. Many diabetics ignore the diet they're supposed to be following until a few days before going in for a blood sugar test. Then they toe the line so the test shows the diabetes to be in good control when in reality it's haywire most of the time. This kind of cheating virtually precludes a cure.

You may find yourself using the excuse that you don't have time to do what the doctor suggests. This reminds us of what exercise therapist Linda Sharp told us about some of her patients. "They have time to hurt," she said with a sigh, "but they don't have the time to do something about it." So when your doctor requires something of you that you feel is too difficult, tiring, or time-consuming, think about whether the time you save is really worth it in pain.

*3. Can you be methodical in your approach and keep good records?* Holism may be unorthodox, but it's not casual or sloppy. Holistic therapies need to be followed as carefully and efficiently as drug therapies or surgical procedures.

You need to be able to report to your doctor with accuracy, even precision—no "I'm-not-sure" or "I-don't-exactly-remember" excuses. To keep everything in order you will have to make extensive notes.

*4. Are you a drug puller?* We came down hard on doctors who push drugs, but we're just as negative about patients who try to pull drugs out of their doctors. Patients have been known to threaten suicide if their doctors won't give them increased dosages of painkillers or tranquilizers. If the doctor refuses and the patient *does* commit suicide, not only is the suicide itself a terrible weight on the doctor's conscience but there's always a pack of hungry lawyers sniffing around to start a malpractice case against him.

Should the doctor yield to the patient's suicide extortion racket and give her the increased dosage, and if, as it well could happen, the patient develops an addiction, the same sniffing-lawyer pack is there ready to start a malpractice suit for *that*.

The poor doctor can't win. And neither can you if you decide to turn yourself into a headache-drug junkie.

5. *Will you try to take advantage of your doctor?* If you call him constantly to discuss every little problem, try to monopolize his time in the office, use him as your father confessor, you're actually taking advantage of your sister sufferers who then can't be fitted into his schedule.

It's ironic but, once you've found a doctor who is willing to listen, you have to be responsible enough to restrain yourself and stick to the facts of your headache problem. Your personal life problems *are* a part of the total picture of your headache, true, but a mention of their existence is enough. A headache specialist is not a psychiatrist and cannot be expected to straighten out your marriage, assuage your guilt feelings, release your inhibitions, or do whatever else is required to give you psychic peace.

If your life problems are weighing unbearably upon you and you feel they are contributing significantly to your headaches, then you should ask your headache specialist to recommend a therapist to help you with them.

6. *Do you really want to get rid of your headaches?* This is the most significant question of all to ask yourself and we hope you aren't offended that we bring it up, although you probably are. In fact, if we were in the room with you now it's likely we'd have to cover our ears from your shoutings of "Of course I do! These headaches are ruining my life. I'd give *anything* to be rid of them."

We believe you, and we're sure you believe yourself. But

it is true that some women subconsciously cling to their headaches. Their headaches fulfill a need. Maybe the headaches are giving them some sort of power over others. One intractable headache sufferer was an older woman who was ignored by her married children except when she was in the throes of one of her excruciating (and *genuine*) "migraine" attacks. Then the children would all cluster solicitously around her. Her doctor believes it is likely she'll remain intractable.

Maybe headaches are getting some women out of something they don't want to do. Along these lines we heard the story—for a change—of a young man who suffered from chronic headaches. He was unmarried, in his early thirties, athletic, good-looking, holding down a responsible job. In answer to the inevitable question of "Why isn't a great guy like you married?" he always replied, "As long as I have these headaches I can *never* get married."

A headache may also be a protection. Dr. Jack Pinsky, a psychiatrist at both City of Hope and Cedars-Sinai explains that sometimes a person senses that without the headache she would have to face up to some other life situation that is too dreadful to contemplate. As long as she has the headache to contend with, she can push that other dark dreadful aside and, like Scarlett O'Hara, think about it tomorrow.

Luckily there is a way to see if you really wholeheartedly want to get rid of your headache pain. You must ask yourself frankly—and answer yourself honestly— whether you are willing to put forth all the time and effort and make the major life changes a cure may require. Or are you going to be too tired, too busy, too sick, too confused, too discouraged, too anything to do it? That, of course, remains to be seen.

## PAYING THE RANSOM

Once you have determined to rid yourself of headaches no matter what the cost, cost becomes a factor to consider. As any long-term headache sufferer knows, the cost of medical help in dollars can be as intense as the pain. Doctors' bills and treatments come high and go higher every year. We might even say without exaggeration that the road to the poorhouse is paved with prescriptions.

There may be no way to keep your chronic headache from being a financial drain, and you have to keep the brain inside your aching head functioning at all costs in order to keep from turning that drain into a disaster. So what do you do?

## Insurance Company Policy

"Oh, but you're lucky. You have medical insurance." That is the way people often dismissed the economic problems of June's disease. Apparently these people have never had to make a claim on a policy—or at least not a claim for something that is not as clear-cut as surgery.

Even when medical insurance carriers, as they call themselves, deign to pay a claim, they pay only a percentage of what *they* consider a "reasonable and customary" fee for the service. No physician practicing since the depth of the 1930s Depression has the same idea of "reasonable and customary" as the insurance companies have. Consequently, you are only paid a percentage of a percentage and that gets you down to the price of peanuts as compared to the price of diamonds.

Of course, even this small recompense is something. Sometimes you get nothing at all. This is particularly true when you're using the newer holistic therapies. Insurance companies are in no hurry to bring additional treatments under the rather leaky umbrella of their coverage, so the headache sufferer often winds up getting soaked. Dr. Bresler told us that about the only way he could help patients collect for holistic treatment would be to hospitalize them. He said that this was not only unnecessary but that a hospital environment would create additional stress for them.

Is there anything that can be done about the situation?

As things now stand there isn't much, but you ought to work on every one of the possibilities that are available to you.

**Persistence.** When asked what was the secret of being a successful writer, Ernest Hemingway responded, "You have to be the world's most persistent sonofabitch." We are of the opinion that the same advice holds true for those who would succeed in getting money out of insurance companies. From our observation, insurance companies derive their grossest profits from people who just give up, figuring that after all their time is worth something. Even if your time *is* worth something, as all of ours is, you still should keep at them. Make it a point of honor and a challenging game to wear them down when your cause is just. You'll not only be helping yourself for now but helping yourself and others in the future.

Don't take no for an answer, and above all don't take no answer for an answer. The modern way for companies to avoid doing what they don't want to do is to ignore you. Be not ignored. If there's a local office, call and call and call again. If there isn't a local office, write registered letters (so they'll notice them) with return receipt requested, so they'll not be able to deny having received your letter. Keep all documentation on your claim. Send only photostats of records so they can't lose the originals.

When every possible appeal has been made to the insurance company—and turned down by them—*still* don't give up. Write to the State Commissioner of Insurance for help, sending along copies of all the documentation of your claim.

Another insurance company ploy is the "it's-not-my-job" gambit. This was what happened to June with her TMJ problem. Her dental insurance didn't recognize the treatment as solving a dental problem, because in the larger sense it didn't. On the other hand, since the work was done by a dentist and was done on the teeth, the medical insurance decided it was not their baby, either. As

June said in one of her myriad letters of protest to the insurance company:

It really seems ironical to me that over the last five years as I sought a cure for my chronic headaches, you have paid out funds to doctor after doctor who misdiagnosed my problem and gave me treatment unrelated to the problem. Now that a specialist in headaches has correctly diagnosed the cause and put me in the care of someone who was capable of giving treatment related to the problem, you want to deny payment. Obviously I am in the classic Catch-22 situation. If according to the professionals on the two sides of the fence, my claim does not qualify as either medical or dental, then what is it? It's certainly not voodoo, though the dramatic results make me think it is.

Miraculously, June's campaign finally worked. She received the standard reimbursement of 80 percent (of $500) for the temporary dental plane. But, again ironically—and illogically—they refused to pay for the permanent work. (Probably because it cost $4,200!) At any rate, two years later, she is still fighting it out. And she's following our advice to you. She's *not giving up*.

**Playing the Claim Game.** The significant items in a successful claim seem to be:

1. Has a claim for this kind of service ever been honored before by another insurance company? When possible submit documentation of this.
2. Was the service rendered by a doctor? Although June received only 50 percent of her claim for the rather unorthodox treatment of acupuncture, she did receive that much because it was done by an M.D. We are certain that had she had acupressure from an unlicensed practitioner, her claim would have been chuckled out of the Medical Review Department. Her group insurance program de-

fines "doctor" very specifically as an M.D., osteopath, dentist, podiatrist, chiropractor, optometrist, psychologist, or Christian Science practitioner. It does not mention hypnotist, biofeedback therapist, acupressurist, or Hindu guru.

3. How is the claim presented by the doctor or therapist? If something new like biofeedback is done in the doctor's office and written up simply as an office visit, it is likely to slip through more easily than if it is given its rightful name. Dr. Greene has learned from experience never to use the phrase "to open the bite" in claims because that causes their nonpaying hackles to rise.

**Financial Safety in Numbers?**

The medical care group concept of medical practice is growing in this country. Sometimes, as it is where we work, you're given an opportunity to join a total coverage plan with a group practice such as Kaiser or Ross-Loos, which takes care of all your medical services at no extra cost to you.

This may seem to be the thriftier route to take. After all, a person suffering idiopathic headaches is always passed around among a lot of different specialists, and all of them are paid for in full with a group practice. In our opinion, though, for a headache sufferer the group plan may not be the bargain it seems, at least not at this stage of development of the art and science of headache-as-a-disease-in-itself treatment.

Most of these medical services simply don't have a headache specialist or pain control unit. They're hard enough to find in private practice. Therefore, if you're on one of these plans either you'll have to waste more time futilely bouncing from internist to otolaryngologist to allergist to whatever or you'll have to do as one of our Valley College headache underground members did: Pay for the headache expert on your own while keeping the health plan for other medical services. This is not an inexpensive way of handling it.

## Bill of Health

One way of keeping the wolf of bankruptcy from your door is to talk frankly with your doctor about the costs of proposed treatments, pointing out (truthfully) what your income is and the difficulty you're going to have in paying for a treatment as expensive as, say, long-term allergy shots or TMJ bite adjustment. Doctors are generally reasonable people who will make financial adjustments when it's possible.

And finally, if the choice is up to you, don't forget the cost savings of the more holistic treatments. The UCLA Pain Control Unit gave this dramatic example: Conventional nonsurgical treatment of low-back pain could cost as much as $5,000 and surgery could run that figure up to $10,000. But acupuncture can often be a more effective treatment and its total cost would be more like $400.

And while you're working toward a clean bill of health, don't forget to give yourself some encouraging words as you set forth on the road to recovery.

# 9

## HEADACHE FOOTNOTE: ON THE ROAD TO RECOVERY

In the book *Zen and the Art of Motorcycle Maintenance*, Robert Pirsig makes the point that "the real cycle you're working on is a cycle called yourself." In your case, the headache mystery you're working on is a mystery called you. And the real mystery is what changes you need to make in your life, because your headache is telling you that changes *do* need to be made. You have been told before by other voices, but you probably didn't listen. The only voice most of us *will* listen to is the voice of physical pain or illness, because those voices cannot be ignored.

Although June's headache was telling her that her bite was out of alignment, it was also telling her that many factors of her life were out of alignment. We're convinced that if she had changed her bite and nothing else, the dam would have spilled over anyway and headaches would have made their persistent demand for changes again.

In fact, about a year after the headaches had been cured, June heard a subtle whisper in the form of the beginnings of congestion behind the bridge of her nose. This happened one particularly stressful diabetes lecturing weekend in San Francisco. We had flown into San Francisco Friday after work and had an hour-long newspaper interview about one of our books, followed by a meeting with nurses, and then dinner with the officers of the diabetes association, followed by the talk and a long question and answer period with an audience of several hundred people. This was all topped off by a sleepless night for both of us because our hotel rooms were next door to the hospitality suite of a convention. The next morning the whisper was heard. June heeded it with a full day of mind-washing and body exercising with long walks. The incipient headache packed up its congestion and stole away.

What kinds of holistic headache crime prevention changes has June made in her life? On a clear-cut practical level, because of her increased body awareness, she has become a semivegetarian (lacto-ovo-fisho with an occasional taste of chicko). She has also permanently incorporated into her life many of the relief and de-stressing techniques that have been most effective for her: yoga, running, Zen meditation, and autogenics.

Have these changes been restrictive? Far from it. Here is a Zen riddle for you. She now creates more time in her life by taking time from it for her holistic practices. As proof of her increased capacity, she is now a librarian and a half, working more than full-time. She never takes a day of sick leave, only an occasional (unpaid) day of *well* leave when she has something important or exciting she wants to do.

June now teems with life force, or as the yogis say, *prana*. This is the person who for five years was the woman in the iron mask of pain, unable to work, unable to play, unable to even visualize a future. Now she can state at age fifty-five, "the best is yet to come" and actually see it happening. She hates to say it out loud and tempt the gods, but she is happy.

## HAPPY TALK

Another happy-ending tale of a holistic cure comes from Norman Cousins, editor of *The Saturday Review*. He was lying in the hospital in agony suffering from a collagen disease that a whole battery of experts couldn't diagnose. One day he accidentally saw a letter his doctor had written to a mutual friend in which appeared the sentence, "I think we're going to lose Norman." That did it. He decided it was time for him to get involved in his own case. He eventually succeeded in curing himself with a combination of massive doses of vitamin C and laughter. Yes, laughter! He discovered that ten minutes of genuine belly laughter (he used video tapes of old Candid Camera TV shows) would give him about two hours of pain-free sleep, and he eventually got rid of the pain and the disease totally.

The laughter half of Norman Cousins' cure should not be dismissed lightly. It was at least as important as the vitamin C and maybe more so.

Dr. Bresler of the UCLA Pain Control Unit once said in a radio interview that the patient's attitude is one of the prime factors in how effective any treatment will be. He wished that he could check a patient's "serum fun level" in the same way that he checks a patient's serum cholesterol level, because those with a high capacity for enjoyment also have a high capacity for pain control. "We want to make sure our patients have enough fun to help them break their negative life attitudes. A person can't experience intense pain at the same time he is experiencing joy."

As you may have noticed we have always tried to keep our sense of humor operative even in the darkest days of headache pain and in our writing about it. One of our life philosophies is to take the light things seriously and the serious things lightly. There is probably nothing more serious in your life than your headache and your search for a cure. Try to take it lightly.

## THE GREAT PRETENDER

But what if you don't feel full of fun and optimism and energy after the months or years of pain behind you and possibly still in front of you? Well then, you just *pretend* you're a happy person.

Kurt Vonnegut had as the moral of his book, *Mother Night*, "We are what we pretend to be, so we must be careful about what we pretend to be." Mark that well. Pretend to be a miserable, down-feeling headachoholic with your joy gland totally atrophied and that's what you'll be. Decide to be a happy, healthy, vital person, and *that's* what you'll be.

Remember that in some of the pain clinics the patients are not allowed to dwell on or even talk about their pain. They have to act like functioning well people. They are rewarded for ignoring their pain. And let us pause here briefly to consider how you reward yourself when you have a headache. Do you let yourself lie down in a darkened room and escape from the pressing duties and heavy demands that daily flatten you out?

If so, maybe you could flip the reward switch to the opposite position. Reward yourself with an afternoon or evening off when you feel especially well. Do something you especially enjoy and never have time for—even if it's just doing nothing. Whatever you do, you'll be practicing a kind of self-conditioning in which your feeling-well state is reinforced by rewards while we may hope your headache state is extinguished.

## HUG THERAPY

For some women a headache is a subconscious cry for love and tender treatment. Because they can't bring themselves to march up to someone and say directly what they really need, they announce a pain (a *real* pain) to elicit the sympathy, the soothing touch they need.

This is why one prescription that Dr. Bresler always

gives his chronic pain patients is four hugs a day. He considers these hugs so important that he even advises his patients who don't have a huggee handy to approach strangers in the supermarket and hug them.

Family therapist Helen Colton would endorse this prescription. In the December 1977 issue of *Forum Magazine* she points out that "our need to be touched is as basic as our need for food. ... Without it we get a kind of malnutrition of the spirit." And one of the symptoms of malnutrition of the spirit can be chronic headaches.

If a hug, a warm human touch is what you need, learn to recognize that need and get it met directly ("I need a hug!"). Then you won't have to use that oblique and painful need-meeting device of a headache.

And while you're hugging and programming yourself for fun and joy and taking general care of your health and living with your pain, never give up the hope that someday soon you may be able to live without it. For no matter how many years your headaches have been with you, no matter how many doctors and remedies you've tried, remember: You have not by any means explored every possibility.

Start exploring. You are no longer helpless. You don't have to be a victim. From this moment on misery is optional.

# APPENDIX A
# GENERIC NAMES OF
# HEADACHE DRUGS

| Brand Name | Generic Name |
|---|---|
| Amytal | Amobarbital |
| Cafergot | Ergotamine with caffeine |
| Darvon | Propoxyphene |
| Deseril | Methysergide maleate |
| Dilatin | Diphenylhydantoin |
| Equavil | Meprobamate |
| Fiorinal | Butalbital compound |
| Gynergen | Ergotamine |
| Librium | Chlordiazepoxide |
| Luminal | Phenobarbital |
| Mellaril | Thioridazine |
| Miltown | Meprobamate |
| Periactin | Cyproheptadine |
| Sansert | Methysergide maleate |
| Talwin | Pentazocine |
| Tempra | Acetominophen |
| Thorazine | Chlorpromazine |
| Tylenol | Acetominophen |
| Valium | Diazepam |

# APPENDIX B
# SAFE FOODS LIST

(Foods generally safe in normally healthy individuals.)

| Vegetables | Fruits | Meat and Poultry |
|---|---|---|
| Artichokes | Apples | Beef |
| Asparagus | Apricots | Chicken |
| Beets | Blueberries | Lamb |
| Broccoli | Cherries | Turkey |
| Carrots | Cranberries | Veal |
| Cauliflower | Dates | |
| Celery | Grapes | **Miscellaneous** |
| Cucumbers | Peaches | Fruit pies |
| Eggplant | Pears | Gelatins |
| Green beans | Raisins | Hamburgers |
| Leafy greens | | (avoid pickles |
| Mushrooms | | and sauces) |
| Parsnips | | |
| Peas | | |
| Potatoes | | |
| Sprouts | | |

Keep diet as balanced as possible. Eat lightly when stressed or tired and be especially careful to avoid salt at these times.

*Used with permission of Dorothy Lindholm.*

# APPENDIX C
# TMJ SPECIALISTS AND CLINICS

**CALIFORNIA**

**Encino**
Arnold R. Greene, D.D.S.
16260 Ventura Boulevard
**La Crescenta**
Douglas H. Morgan, D.D.S.
3043 Foothill Boulevard, Suite 8
**Los Angeles**
Victor W. Mintz, D.D.S.
2080 Century Park East, Suite 1208
Century City

University of Southern California School of Dentistry
TMJ and Peri-Oral Pain Clinic
925 W. 34th Street

**FLORIDA**

**Gainesville**
University of Florida College of Dentistry

## NEW YORK

**New York**
Facial Pain-Temporomandibular Joint Clinic
Columbia University School of Dental & Oral Surgery
630 W. 168th Street

## VIRGINIA

**Falls Church**
National Capital Center for Craniofacial Pain

## WASHINGTON

**Seattle**
School of Dental Medicine
University of Washington

# APPENDIX D
# PAIN CLINICS

**ALABAMA**

**Anniston**
Pain Clinic
1029 Christine
**Birmingham**
University of Alabama
  at Birmingham
19th Street & 6th Ave., S.

**ARIZONA**

**Phoenix**
Surgicenter Pain
  Control Unit
1040 E. McDowell
**Tucson**
Pain Clinic
University of Arizona
1501 N. Campbell Ave.

Veterans Administration
  Hospital

**CALIFORNIA**

**Beverly Hills**
Biofeedback Medical Clinic
9735 Wilshire Blvd.

Beverly Hills Headache
  and Pain Medical Group
Cedars-Sinai
  Medical Tower
8631 W. 3rd St.,
  Suite 1030E
**Carson**
The Chinese Acupuncture
  Therapy for Pain
Carson Medical Center
**Duarte**
Pain Center
City of Hope National
  Medical Center
1500 E. Duarte Rd.
**La Jolla**
Pain Treatment Center
Scripps Clinic Medical
  Institution
10666 N. Torrey Pines Rd.
**Loma Linda**
Pain Control Center
Loma Linda University
  Medical Center
**Los Angeles**
Anesthesiology &
  Pain Management
1300 N. Vermont Ave.

Pain Center
University of California
  at Los Angeles
UCLA School of Medicine
10833 LeConte Ave.

Veterans Administration
  Wadsworth Hospital
11000 Wilshire Blvd.
**Merced**
Louis W. Lewis, M.D.
443 W. 22nd St.
**Mountain View**
El Camino Hospital
2500 Grant Rd.
**North Hollywood**
Pain Control
  Medical Group
7535 Laurel Canyon Blvd.
**Pasadena**
Pain Clinic
Huntington Memorial
  Hospital
100 Congress St.
**Pomona**
Casa Colina Hospital for
  Rehabilitative Medicine
255 E. Bonita Ave.
**San Diego**
Naval Regional
  Medical Center
Balboa Park

Veterans Administration
  Hospital
3350 La Jolla Village Dr.

**San Francisco**
San Francisco Veterans
  Administration Hospital
4150 Clement St.

University of California
  Medical Center
**San Luis Obispo**
Cox Pain Center
2066-B Chorro St.
**Santa Monica**
James Y. P. Chen, M.D.
1304 15th St.
**Torrance**
Pain Clinic
Harbor General Hospital
1000 W. Carson St.

## COLORADO

**Denver**
St. Joseph's Hospital
1835 Franklin

Pain Clinic
University of Colorado
  Medical Center
4200 E. 9th Ave.

## CONNECTICUT

**Greenwich**
Pain Clinic
Greenwich Hospital
Perryridge Rd.

**Middlebury**
Research Institute of
Acupuncture and
  Chinese Medicine
N. Benson Rd.
**West Haven**
Veterans Administration
  Hospital

**DISTRICT OF**
  **COLUMBIA**

Greater Southeast
  Community Hospital
1310 Southern Ave., S.E.

Providence Hospital
1150 Varnum, N.E.

**FLORIDA**

**Gainesville**
Pain Control
Department of
  Anesthesiology
Shands Teaching Hospital
University of Florida

Veterans Administration
  Hospital

**Pensacola**
W. C. Payne Medical
  Arts Building
5149 N. 9th Ave., Suite 307

**St. Petersburg**
Hubert Rutland Hospital
5115 58th Ave., N.

**GEORGIA**

**Atlanta**
Pain Control
Center of Rehabilitation
Emory University
**Marietta**
Atlanta Pain Clinic
2550 Windy Hill Road,
Suite 104

**IDAHO**

**Lewiston**
St. Joseph's Hospital
  Pain Clinic
415 6th St.

**ILLINOIS**

**Chicago**
Central Community
  Hospital
5701 S. Wood St.

Cook County Hospital
1825 W. Harrison St.

Diamond Headache
  Clinic, Ltd.
3321 W. Columbus Ave.

Michael Reese
Medical Center
2929 S. Ellis Ave.

Mount Sinai Hospital
1500 S. Fairfield Ave.

Rush Pain Center
1725 W. Harrison St.,
Suite 262

Schwab Rehabilitation
Hospital
1401 S. California Blvd.

**Downey (Great Lakes)**
North Chicago Veterans
Administration Hospital
**Great Lakes**
U.S. Naval Regional
Medical Center
**Maywood**
Loyola University Hospital
2160 S. 1st Ave.
**Skokie**
R. C. Balagot, M.D. &
Associates, Ltd.
4332 Oakton St.
**Wheaton**
Marianjoy Rehabilitation
Hospital
26 W. 171 Roosevelt Rd.

**INDIANA**

**Elkhart**
Elkhart General Hospital
600 East Blvd.
**Indianapolis**
Community Hospital
Rehabilitation Center
for Pain
1500 N. Ritter Ave.
**South Bend**
St. Joseph's Hospital
811 E. Madison

**IOWA**

**Mason City**
St. Joseph's Mercy Hospital
84 Beaumont Dr.
**Sioux City**
Neurological Institute and
Pain Center, P.C.
809 Badgerow Building

**KENTUCKY**

**Lexington**
Pain Rehabilitation Clinic
University of Kentucky
Medical Center
800 Rose St.
**Louisville**
Pain Clinic
University of Louisville
316 MDR Building,
Health Science Center

Veterans Hospital
Pain Clinic
800 Zorn Ave.

**LOUISIANA**

**Metairie**
New Orleans Pain Clinic
3225 N. Labarre Rd.
**Shreveport**
Doctor's Hospital
Pain Unit
Doctor's Hospital
1130 Louisiana Ave.

**MARYLAND**

**Baltimore**
Pain Treatment Center
Johns Hopkins Hospital
601 N. Broadway St.
**Silver Springs**
Fairland Pain Clinic
13616 Colefair Dr.

**MASSACHUSETTS**

**Boston**
Beth Israel Hospital
330 Brookline Ave.

Pain Service
Massachusetts General
Hospital
Fruit St.

Robert B. Brigham
Hospital
125 Parker Hill Ave.
**Worcester**
Pain Clinic
University of Massachusetts
Medical Center
55 Lake Avenue, N.

**MICHIGAN**

**Ann Arbor**
University of Michigan
Medical Center
**Detroit**
Sinai Hospital of Detroit
6767 W. Outer Dr.
**Lansing**
Ingham Medical Center
Pain Clinic
401 W. Greenlawn
**Southfield**
Detroit Pain Clinic, P.C.
16800 W. 12 Mile Rd.,
Suite 203

Rehabilitation Center
22401 Foster Winter Dr.

**MINNESOTA**

**Mankato**
St. Joseph's Hospital
413 N. 4th St.

**Minneapolis**
Metropolitan Medical
  Center and Waconia
  Ridgeview Hospital
900 S. 8th St.

Minneapolis Pain Clinic
4225 Golden Valley Road

## MISSISSIPPI

**Jackson**
Curtis W. Caine, M.D.
646 Robinhood Rd.

Mississippi University
  Medical Center
2500 N. State St.
**Meridian**
Jeff Anderson Hospital
2124 14th St.

## MISSOURI

**Lewiston**
Victor M. Parisien, MOPA
416 Sabbattus St.

## MONTANA

**Missoula**
Missoula Pain Clinic
Missoula Community
  Hospital
2827 Fort Missoula Rd.

## NEBRASKA

**Omaha**
Nebraska Pain
  Rehabilitation Unit
University of Nebraska
  Medical Center
42nd Street &
  Dewey Ave.

The Pain Clinic
7701 Pacific St.,
  Suite 123

## NEW HAMPSHIRE

**Hanover**
Dartmouth-Hitchcock
  Medical Center
2 Maynard St.

## NEW JERSEY

**Newark**
Pain Clinic
New Jersey Medical
  School & Affiliated
  Hospitals
**Wayne**
North Jersey Anesthesia
  Associates, P.A.
220 Hamburg Turnpike

## NEW YORK

**Binghampton**
Pain Unit
Our Lady of Lourdes
    Hospital
169 Riverside Dr.

**Bronx**
Acupuncture Clinic
Revson Diagnostic Center
Hospital of the
    Albert Einstein
    College of Medicine
1825 Eastchester Rd.

Headache Unit
Montefiore Hospital &
    Medical Center
111 E. 210th St.

**Brooklyn**
Department of
    Anesthesiology
Maimonides Medical
    Center
4802 10th Ave.

**Kenmore**
Duane H. Ducker, D.O.
1133 Colvin Blvd.

**Flushing**
Parsons Acupuncture
    Clinic
Parsons Hospital
35-06 Parsons Blvd.

**Long Island City**
Boulevard Hospital
46-04 31st Ave.

**New York City**
Ivan K. Goldberg, M.D.
123 E. 83rd St.

Pain Program
Hospital for Joint Diseases
    and Medical Center
1919 Madison Ave.

Nerve Block &
    Neurology Clinic
Presbyterian Hospital

Vanderbilt Clinic
    Columbia-Presbyterian
    Medical Center
622 168th St.

**North Tarrytown**
Phelps Memorial Hospital
N. Broadway

**Syracuse**
S.U.N.Y., Upstate
    Medical Center
750 E. Adams St.

**Valhalla**
Pain Clinic
Westchester County
    Medical Center
Grasslands Reservation

# NORTH CAROLINA

**Chapel Hill**
Pain Clinic
University of
 North Carolina
North Carolina Memorial
 Hospital and
 Dental Research Center
**Columbus**
Pain Clinic
Rusk Rehabilitation Center

Pain and Stress
 Treatment Center
Grant Hospital
**Elyria**
Elyria Acupuncture &
 Biofeedback Clinic
100 E. Broad St.,
 Suite 4
**Toledo**
Mercy Hospital
2200 Jefferson Ave.
**Youngstown**
Pain Clinic
St. Elizabeth Hospital
 Medical Center
1044 Belmont Ave.

Youngstown Osteopathic
 Hospital
1319 Florencedale Ave.

# OKLAHOMA

**Tulsa**
Thomas L. Ashcraft, M.D.
 & Associates, Inc.
Doctors' Medical Center

# OREGON

**Portland**
Acupuncture Pain
 Control Center
7227 S.W. Terwilliger

Northwest Pain Center
Woodland Park Hospital
1400 S.E. Umatilla St.

Pain Evaluation Clinic
1120 20th St., N.W.

The Portland Pain Center
Emanuel Rehabilitation
 Center
3001 N. Gantenbein

# PENNSYLVANIA

**Carbondale**
Pain and Acupuncture
 Clinic
141 Salem Ave.

**Clarks Summit**
Willis C. Barnes, M.D.
  Pain Clinic
115 Depot St.
**Drexel Hill**
Pain Clinic-Acupuncture
Delaware County
  Memorial Hospital
Lansdowne &
  Keystone Ave.
**Dubois**
Dubois Hospital
100 Hospital Ave.
**Harrisburg**
Polyclinic Hospital
3rd & Radnor St.
**Johnstown**
Therapeutic and Diagnos-
  tic Pain Clinic
Conemaugh Valley
  Memorial Hospital
1086 Franklin St.
**Latrobe**
Latrobe Nerve Block &
  Pain Studies Clinic
Latrobe Area Hospital
W. 2nd Ave.
**Natrona Heights**
Allegheny Valley Hospital
1300 Carlisle St.
**Philadelphia**
Misericordia Division
Mercy Catholic
  Medical Center
54th Street & Cedar Ave.

Pain Control Center
Temple University Hospital
3401 N. Broad St.

Thomas Jefferson
  University Hospital
1025 Walnut St.
**Pittsburgh**
Pain Control Center
University of Pittsburgh
Presbyterian University
  Hospital
230 Lathrop St.

Shadyside Hospital
5230 Centre Avenue

Veterans Administration
  Hospital
Highland Dr.
**Sayre**
Guthrie Clinic, Ltd.

## RHODE ISLAND

**Providence**
Institute for Behavioral
  Medicine
Summit Medical Center

## SOUTH CAROLINA

**Charleston**
Medical University of
  South Carolina
80 Barre St.

**Columbia**
Richland Memorial
  Hospital
3301 Harden St.

**TENNESSEE**

**Memphis**
Pain Clinic
University of Tennessee
66 N. Pauline

**TEXAS**

**Amarillo**
High Plains Baptist
  Hospital
1200 Wallace Blvd.
**Dallas**
Pain Evaluation and
  Treatment Center
University of Texas Health
  Science Center
5323 Harry Hines Blvd.

Pain Relief Center
  (Division of Texas
  Neurological Institute)
Medical City
7777 Forest Lane,
  Suite 109

Veterans Administration
  Hospital
4500 S. Lancaster Rd.

**Galveston**
St. Mary's Hospital
404 8th St.
**Garland**
Garland Pain Clinic
Memorial Hospital
  of Garland
2300 Marie Curie Blvd.
**Houston**
Anesthesiology Pain Clinic
University of Texas Medical
  School at Houston
6400 W. Cullen St.
**San Antonio**
Wilford Hall Hospital
**Temple**
Scott & White Clinic

**UTAH**

**Bountiful**
W. Lynn Richards, M.D.
480 S. 400 E.

**VIRGINIA**

**Danville**
Memorial Hospital
142 S. Main St.

**WASHINGTON**

**Seattle**
Pain Clinic
Harborview Medical
  Center
325 9th St.

Operant Program for
  Chronic Pain
Department of Rehabili-
  tative Medicine
University Hospital
1959 N.E. Pacific

Pain Clinic
Seattle Veterans
  Administration Hospital
4435 Beacon Ave., S.

Swedish Hospital
  Medical Center
747 Summit

University Hospital
1959 Pacific St., N.E.

Virginia Mason Pain Clinic

**Walla Walla**
Walla Walla General
  Hospital
1025 S. Second Ave.

## WEST VIRGINIA

**Morgantown**
West Virginia University
  Medical Center
**South Charleston**
H. J. Thomas Memorial
  Hospital
4605 MacCorkle Ave., S.W.

## WISCONSIN

**Cudahy**
Trinity Memorial Hospital
5900 S. Lake Dr.
**LaCrosse**
Pain and Health Rehabil-
  itation Center
Route 2, Welsh Conlee
**Madison**
Pain Management
  Unit-Rehabilitative
  Medicine
University of Wisconsin
  Hospitals

Center for Health Sciences
University of Wisconsin
  Neurological
  & Rehabilitation Hospital
**Milwaukee-Wood**
Veterans Administration
  Center
5000 W. National Ave.

## PUERTO RICO

**Rio Piedras**
San Juan Pain Clinic
Calle 6 No. 461, Ext.
  San Agustin

# REFERENCES

Brainard, John B. *Control of Migraine*. New York: W. W. Norton, 1977.

Carrington, Patricia. *Freedom in Meditation*. New York: Anchor Press/Doubleday, 1977.

Cousins, Norman. "Anatomy of an Illness as Perceived by the Patient." *Saturday Review*, 5 May 1977, pp. 4-6.

Diamond, Seymour, and Furlong, William Barry. *More Than Two Aspirin*. Chicago: Follett, 1976.

Easwaran, Eknath. *The Mantram Handbook*. Berkeley, Calif.: Nilgiri Press, 1977.

Friedman, Arnold P., and Frazier, Shervert H., Jr. *The Headache Book*. New York: Dodd, Mead, 1973.

Graedon, Joe. *The People's Pharmacy*. New York: St. Martin's Press, 1976.

Hass, Frederick J., and Dolan, Edward F., Jr. *What You Can Do About Your Headaches*. Chicago: Henry Regnery, 1973.

Hays, K. M. *Do Something About That Migraine*. New York: Award Books, 1968.

Lance, James W. *Headache: Understanding, Alleviation*. New York: Charles Scribner's Sons, 1975.

*Physician's Desk Reference*. 31st ed. Oradell, N.J.: Medical Economics, 1977.

Rainer, Tristine. *The New Diary*. Los Angeles: J. P. Tarcher, 1978.

Shealy, C. Norman. *The Pain Game*. Millbrae, Calif.: Celestial Arts, 1976.

Speer, Frederic. *Migraine*. Chicago: Nelson-Hall, 1977.

Turner, James S. *The Chemical Feast*. New York: Grossman, 1970.

Vonnegut, Kurt. *Mother Night*. New York: Dell, 1966.

# SUGGESTED READING

**AUTOGENICS**
Lindemann, Hannes. *Relieve Tension the Autogenic Way*. New York: Peter H. Wyden, 1973.
Shealy, C. Norman. *90 Days to Self-Health*. New York: Dial, 1977.

**BIOFEEDBACK**
Brown, Barbara B. *Stress and the Art of Biofeedback*. New York: Harper & Row, 1977.
Karlin, M., and Andrews, L. *Biofeedback: Turning On the Power of Your Mind*. New York: Harper & Row, 1977.
Stern, Robert M., and Ray, William J. *Biofeedback: How to Control Your Body, Improve Your Health and Increase Your Effectiveness*. Homewood, Ill.: Dow Jones-Irwin, 1977.

**MEDITATION**
Benson, Herbert. *The Relaxation Response*. New York: William Morrow, 1975.
Bloomfield, Harold; Cain, Michael; and Jaffe, Dennis. *TM: Discovering Inner Energy and Overcoming Stress*. New York: Delacorte, 1975.
Easwaran, Eknath. *Meditation*. Petaluma, Calif.: Nilgiri Press, 1978.
Hittleman, Richard. *Richard Hittleman's Guide to Yoga Meditation*. New York: Bantam Books, 1969.
Suzuki, Shunryu. *Zen Mind, Beginner's Mind*. New York: Weatherhill, 1970.

# RELAXATION AND EXERCISE THERAPIES

Carr, Rachel E. *The Yoga Way to Release Tension*. New York: Coward, McCann & Geoghegan, 1974.

Choudhury, Bikram, with Bonnie Jones Reynolds, *Bikram's Beginning Yoga Class*. Los Angeles: J. P. Tarcher, 1978.

Hittleman, Richard. *Richard Hittleman's 28-Day Exercise Plan*. New York: Bantam Books, 1969.

Jacobson, Edmund. *You Must Relax*. New York: McGraw-Hill, 1962.

Ullyot, Joan. *Women's Running*. Mountain View, Calif.: World Publications, 1976.

# RELIEF MEASURES

Bergson, Anika, and Tuchack, Vladimir. *Zone Therapy*. New York: Pinnacle Books, 1974.

Blate, Michael. *The Natural Healer's Acupressure Handbook: G-Jo Fingertip Technique*. New York: Holt, Rinehart and Winston, 1976.

Chan, Pedro. *Finger Acupressure*. Revised enlarged edition. Los Angeles: Price/Stern/Sloan, 1975.

Irwin, Yukiko. *Japanese Finger Pressure for Energy, Sexual Vitality and Relief From Tension and Pain*. Philadelphia and New York: J. B. Lippincott, 1976.

Kurland, Howard. *Quick Headache Relief Without Drugs*. New York: William Morrow, 1977.

# INDEX